AF769395

PUBLIC HEALTH IN THE 21ST CENTURY

CHINESE HERBS AND HERBAL MEDICINE

ESSENTIAL COMPONENTS, CLINICAL APPLICATIONS AND HEALTH BENEFITS

PUBLIC HEALTH IN THE 21ST CENTURY

Additional books in this series can be found on Nova's website under the Series tab.

Additional e-books in this series can be found on Nova's website under the e-book tab.

PUBLIC HEALTH IN THE 21ST CENTURY

CHINESE HERBS AND HERBAL MEDICINE

ESSENTIAL COMPONENTS, CLINICAL APPLICATIONS AND HEALTH BENEFITS

BRIAN L. DUKE
EDITOR

New York

Copyright © 2015 by Nova Science Publishers, Inc.

All rights reserved. No part of this book may be reproduced, stored in a retrieval system or transmitted in any form or by any means: electronic, electrostatic, magnetic, tape, mechanical photocopying, recording or otherwise without the written permission of the Publisher.

For permission to use material from this book please contact us:
nova.main@novapublishers.com

NOTICE TO THE READER

The Publisher has taken reasonable care in the preparation of this book, but makes no expressed or implied warranty of any kind and assumes no responsibility for any errors or omissions. No liability is assumed for incidental or consequential damages in connection with or arising out of information contained in this book. The Publisher shall not be liable for any special, consequential, or exemplary damages resulting, in whole or in part, from the readers' use of, or reliance upon, this material. Any parts of this book based on government reports are so indicated and copyright is claimed for those parts to the extent applicable to compilations of such works.

Independent verification should be sought for any data, advice or recommendations contained in this book. In addition, no responsibility is assumed by the publisher for any injury and/or damage to persons or property arising from any methods, products, instructions, ideas or otherwise contained in this publication.

This publication is designed to provide accurate and authoritative information with regard to the subject matter covered herein. It is sold with the clear understanding that the Publisher is not engaged in rendering legal or any other professional services. If legal or any other expert assistance is required, the services of a competent person should be sought. FROM A DECLARATION OF PARTICIPANTS JOINTLY ADOPTED BY A COMMITTEE OF THE AMERICAN BAR ASSOCIATION AND A COMMITTEE OF PUBLISHERS.

Additional color graphics may be available in the e-book version of this book.

Library of Congress Cataloging-in-Publication Data

ISBN: 978-1-63482-085-1
Library of Congress Control Number: 2015930864

Published by Nova Science Publishers, Inc. † New York

Contents

Preface

Radix Bupleuri (Chai Hu) is one of the most commonly used herbs in the Chinese medicine clinical practice. In Chinese medicine, it is believed that Radix Bupleuri is acrid, cool and bitter and enters liver and gallbladder meridians. This book discusses the use of Chinese herbs, such as Chai Hu, and other different herbal medicines for diseases and illnesses such as atopic dermatitis, and for cutaneous wound healing. It discusses the essential components, clinical applications and health benefits of herbal medicine.

Chapter I – A cutaneous wound is a break in the skin integrity as a result of physical, thermal or chemical injuries. There are many types of wounds, such as incisions, lacerations, contusions and burns. After hemostasis occurs at the moment of injury, the wound healing process proceeds to subsequent yet overlapping stages, namely inflammatory, proliferative and remodeling phases. The inflammatory phase consists of phagocytosis and microvascular changes induced by chemical mediators. The proliferative phase mainly involves angiogenesis, granulation tissue formation, wound contraction and re-epithelialization. In the remodeling phase, new collagen formation occurs to strengthen the wound. In general, the strategy for wound care management is to prevent infection and to promote healing. Currently, herbal medicine has increasingly become a field of interest for wound care. A number of investigations into its therapeutic roles in wound management have been conducted in human and animal models. The well-recognized and most studied medicinal plants include *Aloe vera*, *Centella asiatica* and *Curcuma longa.* These herbs have been used for centuries in traditional Chinese medicine and Ayurveda. Based on the existing scientific evidence, the above-mentioned herbal medicines can accelerate cutaneous wound healing and repair by suppressing inflammation, promoting angiogenesis, inducing cellular growth and proliferation, reducing oxidative stress in the wound, controlling infection, and improving wound remodeling. This chapter will provide insight into the mechanisms underlying various stages of cutaneous wound healing. To establish a foundation of basic knowledge, the first part of the chapter provides an overview of wound healing mechanisms, wound management strategies, and experimental approaches to wound healing, including research models for wounding and the evaluation of critical events during each phase of the wound healing process. Also, a wound microcirculation study using a dorsal skinfold chamber preparation and an intravital microscopic technique to demonstrate cutaneous microvascular changes *in vivo* will be described.

Chapter II – Radix Bupleuri (Chai Hu) is one of the most commonly used herbs in the Chinese medicine clinical practice. In Chinese medicine, it is believed that Radix Bupleuri (Chai Hu) is acrid, cool and bitter and enters Liver and Gallbladder meridians. It is used to reduce fever, release the stagnation of Liver Qi and raise clear Yang. Details of its actions, indications, contraindications, dosage and control are discussed from Chinese medicine perspective. In Western medicine, the clinical and experimental studies have shown that Radix Bupleuri (Chai Hu) has anti-inflammatory, antimicrobial, antiviral, immune-regulatory and anti-tumour effects. Radix Bupleuri (Chai Hu) also has effects on central nervous system, cardiovascular system, digestive system and metabolism. This monograph presents details of its pharmacodynamics, pharmacokinetics and mechanism, toxicology and interactions as well as side effects with evidence from comprehensive literature search. Guidelines for its use and regulatory control in different countries are also reviewed.

Chapter III – Atopic dermatitis (AD) is a common chronic inflammatory skin disease in children that could adversely affect their quality of life, and its prevalence is increasing in the last few decades. As definitive cure is lacking, there has been a considerable interest on using traditional Chinese Herbal Medicines (CHM) as an alternative treatment for AD. However, no data are available to provide an overview of the use of CHM for AD. In this chapter, we explored all the available relevant literatures on the clinical applications of CHM for AD, including its indications, contraindications, individual medicines, formulae, regimes, effectiveness, efficacy, safety, adverse effects and toxicity. The main objective is to review the available clinical studies on CHM for its therapeutic use in AD patients and the potential adverse outcomes. Over 140 literatures were identified, including the observational designed studies (exploratory studies, descriptive studies and analytical studies as case series, cohort studies, case-control studies, cross-sectional studies), the experimental studies (quasi- and randomized controlled trials) and the qualitative studies. Based on the principles and workflows from Centre for Evidence-Based Medicine of Oxford University and Cochrane Review, only few studies were selected for the systematic review and further meta-analysis. The result showed that compared with modern medicine groups, combined use of CHMs and modern medicines was significantly effective as a treatment option for atopic dermatitis. However there was insufficient proof on its safety although no specific safety problem was reported in the clinical trials. More scientific evidences through comprehensive studies on the efficacy and safety of CHM for AD are still necessary for its wider application.

In: Chinese Herbs and Herbal Medicine
Editor: Brian L. Duke

ISBN: 978-1-63482-085-1
© 2015 Nova Science Publishers, Inc.

Chapter I

Herbal Medicine and Mechanisms for Cutaneous Wound Healing

Juraiporn Somboonwong, M.D., M.Sc., Dip. Derm.
Department of Physiology, Faculty of Medicine,
Chulalongkorn University, Bangkok, Thailand

Abstract

A cutaneous wound is a break in the skin integrity as a result of physical, thermal or chemical injuries. There are many types of wounds, such as incisions, lacerations, contusions and burns. After hemostasis occurs at the moment of injury, the wound healing process proceeds to subsequent yet overlapping stages, namely inflammatory, proliferative and remodeling phases. The inflammatory phase consists of phagocytosis and microvascular changes induced by chemical mediators. The proliferative phase mainly involves angiogenesis, granulation tissue formation, wound contraction and re-epithelialization. In the remodeling phase, new collagen formation occurs to strengthen the wound. In general, the strategy for wound care management is to prevent infection and to promote healing. Currently, herbal medicine has increasingly become a field of interest for wound care. A number of investigations into its therapeutic roles in wound management have been conducted in human and animal models. The well-recognized and most studied medicinal plants include *Aloe vera*, *Centella asiatica* and *Curcuma longa*.

These herbs have been used for centuries in traditional Chinese medicine and Ayurveda.

Based on the existing scientific evidence, the above-mentioned herbal medicines can accelerate cutaneous wound healing and repair by suppressing inflammation, promoting angiogenesis, inducing cellular growth and proliferation, reducing oxidative stress in the wound, controlling infection, and improving wound remodeling. This chapter will provide insight into the mechanisms underlying various stages of cutaneous wound healing. To establish a foundation of basic knowledge, the first part of the chapter provides an overview of wound healing mechanisms, wound management strategies, and experimental approaches to wound healing, including research models for wounding and the evaluation of critical events during each phase of the wound healing process. Also, a wound microcirculation study using a dorsal skinfold chamber preparation and an intravital microscopic technique to demonstrate cutaneous microvascular changes *in vivo* will be described.

Introduction

A cutaneous wound is a disruption of the normal continuity of the skin caused by a physical, thermal or chemical injury. Cutaneous wounds can be classified into several types according to the character and cause of the injury: incisions, lacerations, contusions and burns.

An incised wound is a wound that is inflicted by a cutting instrument and that involves minimal tissue damage. A lacerated wound is one in which the tissues are torn or mangled by a dull or blunt instrument.

Another injury that results from blunt trauma is called a contusion, in which the skin is unbroken, but the underlying tissues and blood vessels are damaged. Abrasions are associated with a loss of the superficial layer of the skin. Burns can be caused by thermal (heat), electrical, radioactive, or chemical injuries that destroy cellular proteins and cause cell death.

In response to tissue injury, the body restores the continuity and function of the disrupted skin by undergoing wound healing processes that consist of successive albeit overlapping stages. Any alterations during each healing stage can give rise to delayed- or non-healing wounds. Successful healing thus requires a proper treatment regimen, which involves systemic support and local wound care. Since ancient times, herbal medicine has been implicated in the treatment and management of wounds, particularly in the primary healthcare systems of many countries. The role of herbal medicine in wound healing has also gained increasing attention in research.

The objective of this chapter is to provide insight into the mechanisms of action of herbal medicines in wound healing.

The first part of this chapter provides a general consideration of wound healing, and it is intended to describe the basic concepts of wound healing physiology, as well as influential factors, strategies for wound care management, and a brief outline of the associated experimental approaches, including research models and techniques used to evaluate the process of wound healing with an emphasis on the wound microcirculation studies. The aforementioned knowledge is fundamental to provide the scientific evidence needed to clarify the therapeutic efficacy and underlying mechanisms of herbal medicines in wound healing. To achieve this goal, the last part of this chapter provides a compilation of the scientific evidence regarding the therapeutic roles and mechanisms of action of the three most commonly studied medicinal herbs in wound management: *Aloe vera, Centella asiatica,* and *Curcuma longa.*

Part I: General Considerations of Wound Healing Physiology of Wound Healing

Wound healing is a process of the restoration of integrity to injured tissue as the body attempts to cure itself. Tissue injury generally has two outcomes -- regeneration and repair --- depending on the extent and continuity of the injury, as well as the regenerative potential of the affected tissue.

Regeneration is the replacement of the injured tissue by parenchymal cells of the same cell type without significant scar formation, as in moderate sunburn. Repair is replacement with connective tissue, resulting in scarring and fibrosis, as in abscess formation. An understanding of the physiology of wound healing and the factors that affect healing will provide the basis for proper wound care and management.

A number of interrelated physiological mechanisms are implicated in wound healing. After hemostasis occurs at the moment of injury, wound healing generally proceeds to three subsequent yet overlapping stages, namely the inflammatory, proliferative and remodeling phases. After being triggered by tissue injury, these processes involve a complex series of events that are regulated by many cell types and by the mediators produced (Table 1).

Following skin injury, vascular damage is often present that allows the blood to extravasate into the wound.

The body immediately responds to stop the bleeding and to prevent further blood loss via a process called hemostasis. This brief hemostatic period consists of three key events: 1) vasoconstriction; 2) platelet activation and aggregation; and 3) coagulation or clot formation. The first response of the blood vessels to direct injury is vascular smooth muscle constriction, which helps to control bleeding. In endothelial injuries, exposed collagen fibrils underlying the endothelial layer stimulate platelets to adhere to the damaged site. The activated platelets release cytoplasmic granules containing serotonin, which is a vasoconstrictor, and adenosine diphosphate and thromboxane A_2 (TXA2), which trigger platelet aggregation and thus the formation of a temporary platelet plug. The final hemostatic mechanism, i.e., the coagulation or clotting cascade, is initiated by factors that are released from the damaged tissue and activated platelets. This process leads to the conversion of prothrombin into thrombin and, subsequently, fibrinogen into fibrin, which combines with von Willebrand factor and platelets to form a mesh, giving rise to a blood clot [1].

In addition to playing a central role in hemostasis, platelets produce several growth factors and cytokines that regulate the ensuing healing cascade by modulating the functions of leukocytes, endothelial cells and fibroblasts. These platelet-derived molecules include platelet-derived growth factor (PDGF), insulin-like growth factor-1 (IGF-1), epidermal growth factor (EGF), transforming growth factor-beta (TGF-beta), and platelet factor-IV [1-3].

Inflammatory Phase

The inflammatory phase occurs during days 1 to 3 after wound infliction. This phase consists mainly of two components: microvascular changes; and leukocyte recruitment and activation to kill microorganisms via phagocytosis.

These inflammatory reactions are responsible for the characteristic manifestations of inflammation, which are warmth, erythema (redness), edema (swelling), and pain. Inflammation that occurs during this phase is intended to protect against wound infection and to initiate the repair process [2].

Microvascular Changes

Microvascular changes during inflammation include vasodilatation and increased vascular permeability. After temporary vasoconstriction as an immediate response during hemostasis, vasodilatation occurs within seconds to a few minutes.

This process is caused by a vasoconstriction-mediated reduction of blood flow, creating tissue hypoxia, which stimulates the production of vasodilator substances, such as nitric oxide, adenosine, and vasoactive metabolites.

Mast cells also release histamine and other active amines, which cause vasodilatation and increased vascular permeability. Moreover, there is an activation of vasoactive substances, such as serotonin, bradykinin and prostaglandins. Vasodilatation leads to increased blood flow, resulting in erythema and warmth. Increasing vascular permeability results in the leakage of plasma and proteins, producing exudate and edema.

These vascular reactions help to deliver leukocytes and plasma proteins to the injured site. It is worth noting that a proper amount of exudate aids the healing process by cleansing the wound, maintaining a moist environment and facilitating epithelialization [2].

Leukocyte Recruitment and Activation

During leukocyte recruitment and activation, leukocytes are recruited from the circulation to the wound site. Subsequently, they are activated to eliminate microbes and dead tissues.

The mechanisms underlying leukocyte recruitment from the blood vessels to the extravascular space at the focus of the injury involve four steps: 1) margination and rolling along the vessel wall; 2) adhesion of leukocytes to the endothelial surface; 3) transmigration through the endothelium, or diapedesis; and 4) movement toward the site (also called chemotaxis).

These steps are mediated by different molecules: selectins in rolling, such as E-selectin, P-selectin and L-selectin; integrins in adhesion, such as intercellular cell adhesion molecule-1 (ICAM-1) and vascular cell adhesion molecule-1 (VCAM-1), together with integrin activation by chemokines, such as tumor necrosis factor-alpha (TNF-alpha) and interleukin-1 (IL-1); platelet endothelial cell adhesion molecule (PECAM-1; also known as CD31) in transmigration; and chemotactic molecules in chemotaxis, such as chemokines and leukotrienes. Early cellular infiltrates consist predominantly of polymorphonuclear leukocytes or neutrophils within the first 24 to 48 hours. Later, within 48 to 72 hours, circulating monocytes, attracted by molecules derived from platelets and damaged cells, constitute the next cell type to enter the wound and differentiate into tissue macrophages [2].

When recruited to the wound site, leukocytes are activated by several mediators. During the early inflammatory phase, the activated neutrophils ingest bacteria and tissue debris via a process called phagocytosis, and they kill and degrade these microorganisms by releasing lysosomal enzymes, nitric oxide and reactive oxygen species as a result of the oxidative burst that occurs during robust neutrophil activity. In addition, neutrophils can destroy microbes and dead tissues extracellularly by producing these substances, as well as "traps". Therefore, the main function of neutrophils is to prevent infection [2].

During the late phase of the inflammatory process, prior to the proliferative phase, acute inflammation must be terminated, and leukocytes produce anti-inflammatory mediators to limit the reaction. This process is followed by resolution and then initiation of the subsequent repair process. Once activated, macrophages phagocytose any remaining bacteria or debris, and they release proteolytic enzymes to clear the wound site. They also initiate and regulate the subsequent repair process by producing many growth factors that are essential for the proliferation of fibroblasts, smooth muscle cells and endothelial cells. Thus, alterations in macrophage function can lead to impaired healing [2].

Proliferative Phase

Following the cessation of inflammation, the proliferative phase begins approximately by day 3, and it lasts until week 2 to 4 post-wounding, depending on the size of the wound. This phase mainly involves angiogenesis, granulation tissue formation, wound contraction and re-epithelialization.

As such, the mechanisms underlying healing during this stage are designed to restore the vascularization of the wounded area, repair the tissue defect, decrease the wound size and cover the wound surface.

Angiogenesis

The establishment of a vascular supply to the wounded skin, called angiogenesis or neovascularization, is critical for healing. It is the process of new blood vessel development.

Endothelial cells are the key cells in this process, which is stimulated by tissue hypoxia and by a number of growth factors. As mentioned previously, the wounded area is hypoxic, inducing macrophages to release angiogenic growth factors, the most important of which are vascular endothelial growth factor (VEGF) and basic fibroblast growth factor (bFGF or so called FGF-2). New capillary buds or sprouts are then formed from the intact vessels, and they further develop the capillary loop into the wound.

Granulation Tissue Formation

The development of granulation tissue begins approximately 3-5 days post-injury. Granulation tissue consists of newly formed collagen, elastin and capillary networks, and it is characterized by pinkish/red colored moist tissue.

Granulation tissue is formed to provide mechanical support, control cell proliferation, provide a scaffold for tissue renewal, and establish the wound environment. This process is achieved by the action of fibroblasts, which synthesize and deposit extracellular matrix (ECM).

This temporary ECM is composed of collagens (primarily type III collagen) and elastins, proteoglycans and hyaluronic acid, adhesive glycoproteins and adhesion receptors, such as fibronectin, laminin and integrins. The growth factors involved in fibroblast recruitment and activation, as well as ECM deposition, include TGF-beta, PDGF, FGF, and pro-inflammatory cytokines (IL-1 and IL-13). Collagen synthesis is particularly essential for the tensile strength of wounds. Normally, the skin incision develops approximately 20% of the strength of the unwounded skin by the end of 2 weeks and a maximum of 80% at the end of the repair process.

Wound Contraction

Wound contraction begins approximately 7 days after wounding, progressing at a rate of 0.60-0.75 mm/day and usually ceasing by 4-6 months. Contractile forces within the wounds are mediated by the interaction of actin and myosin, which are the cytoplasmic microfilaments of myofibroblasts, and by the interaction between fibroblasts and the ECM. This process is regulated by several growth factors, such as PDGF, TGF-beta and bFGF.

Re-Epithelialization

Re-epithelialization is characterized by epidermal migration to reestablish epithelial continuity. This process is stimulated by EGF and transforming growth factor-alpha (TGF-alpha), which are produced by platelets, macrophages and epidermal cells (also called keratinocytes).

Within 12 to 24 hours after injury, keratinocytes in the basal layer of the epidermis begin to proliferate and migrate centripetally from the wound edges across the wound bed, until the opposite edges touch one another.

In the denuded epidermis, hair follicles constitute the primary source of the re-epithelialization process.

Remodeling Phase

The remodeling phase, which is the final stage of wound healing process, starts one week after wounding and continues over several weeks to 2 years. The synthesis and degradation of collagen occurs simultaneously with the remodeling of new connective tissues. The fibroblast density and capillary growth are reduced over time. The aim of this phase is to provide strength to the wound.

Collagen Turnover and Maturation

Collagen and other ECM components are degraded by matrix metalloproteinases (MMPs), which are a family of metalloenzymes that are produced by neutrophils, macrophages and fibroblasts. MMPs include interstitial collagenases, gelatinases and stromelysins. The synthesis and secretion of these enzymes are regulated by growth factors, cytokines and other agents, and their activity depends on the presence of zinc ions. The result of this process is remodeling of the scar as smaller type III collagen fibers are replaced with thicker collagen fibers that are rich in type I collagen, which is similar to the unwounded tissue, together with the crosslinking of newly formed collagen. As remodeling progresses, the activity of MMPs decreases, while that of the tissue inhibitors of metalloproteinases (TIMPs) produced by most mesenchymal cells increases.

Special Characteristics of Cutaneous Wound Healing

In cutaneous wounds with apposed edges, as in clean, incised wounds with sutures and minimal tissue loss, healing is accomplished via a primary union, or so-called healing by first or primary intention. The prevailing characteristic of the repair process is epithelial regeneration with small scar formation and minimal wound contraction.

However, in wounds with separated edges and considerable tissue loss, healing via secondary intention or secondary union is required. This form of healing principally involves extensive cell proliferation, granulation tissue and wound contraction, eventually leaving a large scar. Burns have a somewhat different pathophysiology and mechanism of healing than incision or excision wounds. Thermal injury, the most common cause of burns, results in more extensive vascular damage, both at the site of injury and to the surrounding area, as well as a pronounced acute inflammatory response.

Following a burn injury, rapid local edema formation occurs, peaking at 1 to 3 hours. This phenomenon is followed by a period of no reflow and resulting tissue ischemia and necrosis, the worst of which are observed at 12 to 24 hours. Subsequently, there is a period of transformation to permit leukocyte and platelet recruitment to the wound site, followed by a phase of wound repair. There can be heavy wound colonization with Gram-positive bacteria in the first 48 hours post-burn.

In hospitalized patients with burn injuries, Gram-positive (*Staphylococcus aureus, Staphylococcus pyogenes*) and Gram-negative bacteria (*Pseudomonas aeruginosa, Escherichia coli*) are common causes of wound infection during the first and second weeks, respectively.

Burn wounds can be classified into three degrees according to the depth of injury. First-degree or superficial-thickness burns, such as sunburns, are limited to the epidermis and are characterized by erythema with or without edema, likely followed by desquamation or peeling. The wound heals rapidly, in 3 to 7 days, without the formation of a scar. Second-degree or partial-thickness burns affect the epidermis and some dermal layers, and they can be classified based on the dermal involvement. Superficial partial-thickness burns involve the upper layers of the dermis.

The prominent features of such burns are erythema and clear blistering derived from edema formation and fluid accumulation at the dermo-epidermal junction. This type of burn usually heals within 2 weeks and leaves a minimal scar. A deep partial-thickness burn involves the deeper layers of the dermis and might or might not form blisters but often produces eschar. Scarring can occur. The average healing time for this type of burn is 2 to 4 weeks.

In a third-degree or full-thickness burn, all of the skin layers, as well as skin appendages such as hair follicles and sweat glands, are damaged. Hypertrophic scarring and contractures always occur.

Factors/Conditions That Affect Wound Healing

Optimal body responses, in terms of order, duration and magnitude, during each phase of the wound healing process are required for successful wound repair.

Table 1. Wound healing mechanisms

Phase and days post-wounding	Key aims	Physiological events	Mediators/cytokines/growth factors
Hemostasis (immediate)	To stop bleeding	Vasoconstriction	Ang II, ET-1, TXA2
		Platelet activation and aggregation	PAF
		Coagulation or clot formation	PAI
Inflammation (days 1-3)	To prevent wound infection and initiate the repair process	Microvascular changes Vasodilatation Increased vascular permeability	Histamine, serotonin, kinins, arachidonic acid metabolites (PGs and LTs), PAF, NO
		Leukocyte recruitment (margination and rolling, leukocyte adhesion, diapedesis, chemotaxis) and activation	Cytokines, chemokines, complements
		Neutrophil infiltration	PDGF, GCSF
		Macrophage infiltration	PDGF, TGF-beta
Proliferation (day 3 to week 2)	To provide mechanical support, control cell proliferation, provide a scaffold for tissue renewal, and establish the wound environment	Angiogenesis to develop new capillaries from endothelial cells	VEGF, FGF, HGF, PDGF, TGF-beta
		Granulation tissue formation Fibroblast proliferation	FGF, PDGF, IL-1, IGF-1, TNF-alpha, HGF, TGF-alpha, EGF, GM-CSF, TGF-beta
		ECM synthesis and deposition	TGF-beta, PDGF, FGF, IGF-1, IL-1, IL-13, TNF-alpha
		Wound contraction, mainly via the action of myofibroblasts	PDGF, bFGF, TGF-beta
		Re-epithelialization originating from keratinocytes and hair follicles	KGF, EGF, bFGF, TGF-alpha, GM-CSF, HGF
Remodeling (week 1 to several weeks)	To provide strength to the wound	Synthesis and degradation of collagen	MMPs, TIMPs
		Reduced fibroblast density	
		Reduced capillary growth	

Ang II, angiotensin II; bFGF, basic fibroblast growth factor; ECM, extracellular matrix; EGF, epithelial growth factor; ET-1, endothelin-1; FGF, fibroblast growth factor; GCSF, granulocyte colony-stimulating factor; GM-CSF, granulocyte-macrophage colony-stimulating factor; HGF, hepatocyte growth factor; IGF-1, insulin-like growth factor-1; IL-1, interleukin-1; IL-13, interleukin-13; LTs, leukotrienes; MMPs, matrix metalloproteinases; NO, nitric oxide; PAF, platelet-activating factor; PAI, plasminogen activator inhibitor; PDGF, platelet-derived growth factor; PGs, prostaglandins; TGF-alpha, transforming growth factor-alpha; TGF-beta, transforming-growth factor-beta; TIMPs, tissue inhibitors of metalloproteinases; TNF-alpha, tumor necrosis factor-alpha; TXA2, thromboxane-A2; VEGF, vascular endothelial growth factor.

However, a number of host factors can modify the quality or adequacy of this process. These factors will be discussed as local and systemic factors that can promote or impair wound healing.

Local Factors

Infection

Infection is considered to be the most important local factor that delays the process of healing in clinical practice [2]. The pathophysiology of delayed wound healing caused by infection is illustrated in Figure 1. When infection occurs locally at the wound site or progresses to invasive systemic infection, increased production of pro-inflammatory cytokines is prolonged, thus extending the inflammatory phase period of the healing process. This extension also leads to an increased level of MMPs, as well as a decreased level of protease inhibitors, causing degradation of the ECM and growth factors, respectively.

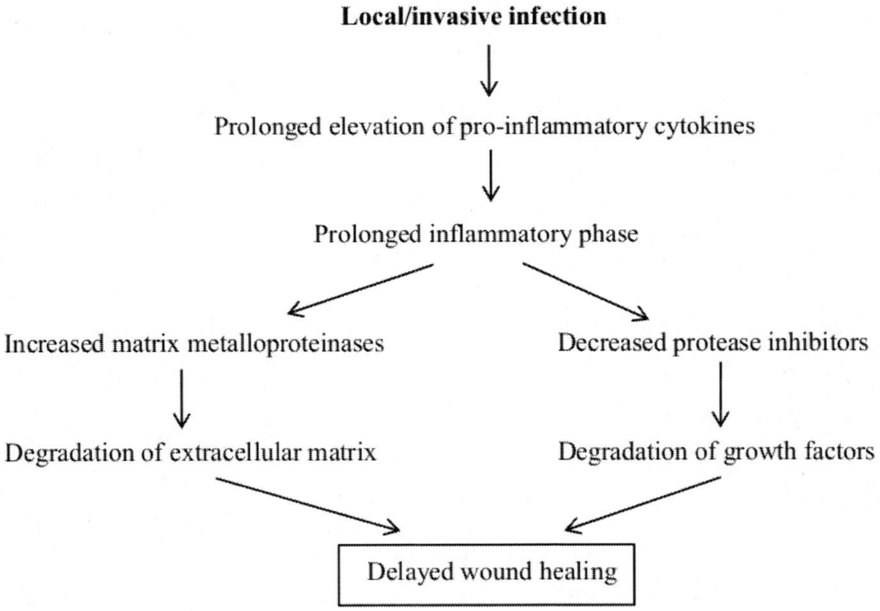

Figure 1. Pathophysiology of delayed wound healing caused by infection.

Additionally, infection increases local tissue destruction caused by bacterial growth and enhances the actions of proteolytic enzymes. As a result, the wound becomes chronic and can fail to heal [4]. Bacteria that are commonly found to infect wounds are *S. aureus, P. aeruginosa* and beta-hemolytic streptococci [4, 5]. These bacteria are also capable of secreting an extracellular polysaccharide matrix to form biofilms, which help to protect them against phagocytosis [5].

Oxygenation

Oxygen plays a pivotal role throughout the healing process, particularly during the inflammatory and proliferative phases. Initially following infliction, all wounds are deficient in oxygen, i.e., in a hypoxic state, which acts as a stimulus for the release of growth factors and angiogenesis [6]. Chronic hypoxia, however, does not enable effective healing, and oxygen is required to continue this process [7]. Given that oxygen is essential for energy production and thus cellular functions, it supports the activities of neutrophils, fibroblasts, macrophages and keratinocytes. Evidence has suggested that adequate tissue oxygen tension levels of no less than 30 to 40 mm Hg are required for the bactericidal action of neutrophils [8], the ability of fibroblasts to synthesize collagen [9] and the angiogenic activity of macrophages [10].

Vascularization

Vascularization of the wounded area is a key factor in the healing process because adequate tissue oxygenation is provided. Therefore, an impaired blood supply retards wound healing, as observed in patients with pressure sores, arterial occlusions or systemic diseases, such as diabetes mellitus. Delayed healing is also a problem for people suffering from venous insufficiency, such as with varicose veins. Obstructed venous drainage gives rise to venous hypertension, which in turn impedes arterial inflow, thereby diminishing oxygen diffusion from the capillaries to the surrounding tissues [11].

Hydration of the Wound Surface

Conservation of hydration at the wound surface can enhance epidermal cell migration and epithelialization [12]. It has been shown that cutaneous wounds with occlusive dressings heal more rapidly than air-exposed wounds, in which dry crust and debris are created to impede epidermal migration [13].

In addition to increased re-epithelialization, moist wound healing has many advantages, including decreases in dehydration and cell death, reductions in wound infection and pain, and increases in angiogenesis and autolytic debridement [14-17].

Mechanical Variables

A variety of mechanical variables can have adverse effects on wound healing. The presence of foreign bodies, such as wood, glass, metal, suture material and debris, can lead to wound infections. A crust prevents epithelial migration. A hematoma reduces repair and tensile strength and also subjects wounds to infection.

In addition, increased tension at the wound edges decreases the rate of healing, wound contraction and wound strength and likely causes wound dehiscence [18].

Ionizing Radiation

Wounds that are exposed to ionizing radiation heal slowly because the irradiation not only inhibits cell proliferation but also injures keratinocytes, fibroblasts, and the appendages to and vasculature of the skin. This damage results in altered wound contraction, poor granulation tissue formation and decreased wound strength [18].

Systemic Factors

Age and Sex

Wound healing is compromised in the elderly. With advancing age, normal skin exhibits changes that have potentially adverse effects on healing, such as decreases in the number of fibroblasts, mast cells and macrophages, diminished collagen content and impaired microcirculation.

There are also age-related alterations in all phases of the healing process. During hemostasis and the inflammatory phase, enhanced platelet aggregation and increased secretion of inflammatory mediators occur, leading to an early excessive inflammatory response.

During the proliferative phase, re-epithelialization, angiogenesis and collagen formation are delayed. In the final phase of wound healing, the remodeling phase, collagen turnover and remodeling are reduced, producing delayed and decreased wound strength. It is currently accepted that the impact of aging on wound healing is mainly a time delay, but in healthy elderly individuals, the overall quality of healing is not markedly impaired *per se* [19].

The effects of age-related changes on normal and wounded skin are profound when coupled with extrinsic factors, such as co-existing medical conditions.

Sex is another factor that influences wound healing during aging. Studies indicate that elderly men have a slower rate of healing than elderly women. Androgens negatively affect cutaneous wound healing, whereas estrogen can reverse the decline in healing in both aged men and women [20]. This phenomenon is partially due to the roles of estrogen in the regulation of cutaneous wound healing due to genes associated with inflammation, protease inhibition, epidermal function, regeneration and matrix production [21].

Nutrition

Nutrition has long been considered an important factor that affects wound healing. Malnutrition, which can be caused by decreased intake, trauma or major surgery, results in the failure of wounds to heal. Under such conditions, nutritional support with proper intake of energy, as well as macro- and micronutrients, has been recognized as an effective measure for healing.

Macronutrients that play significant roles in the healing process include carbohydrates, fat, proteins, and amino acids, such as arginine and glutamine. Carbohydrates and fats are utilized as sources of energy for the cells involved in capillary formation and collagen deposition [22]. Protein is very critical for collagen production, neovascularization, fibroblast proliferation, wound remodeling and immune functions [23, 24]. Arginine facilitates wound healing [25] because it is a precursor to proline, which is an integral component of collagen, and to nitric oxide, which regulates collagen formation, cell proliferation and wound contraction [26]. Glutamine has been shown to stimulate the inflammatory response [27] and to enhance wound strength [28].

Several micronutrients also benefit wound repair. These nutrients include vitamins A, C, E and trace elements, such as zinc, copper, iron and magnesium. Vitamin C functions as a cofactor in the hydroxylation of proline and lysine for collagen synthesis. Vitamin C also improves immune functions by facilitating leukocyte migration into wounds, thus increasing resistance to wound infection. In addition, vitamin C is important for the inflammatory phase of wound healing, and it helps to prevent molecular damage through its anti-inflammatory and antioxidant effects [29, 30]. Similarly, vitamins A and E possess anti-inflammatory and antioxidant properties. Vitamin A also promotes re-epithelialization, the synthesis of collagen and hyaluronate, and immune responses [31-33]. Nonetheless, excessive vitamin A can also delay healing [34]. In animal studies, vitamin E has been reported to enhance wound repair [27, 33]. This effect, however, has not yet been validated in clinical studies [35]. Similar to vitamin A, high doses of vitamin E can negatively affect wound healing [36].

Zinc is a cofactor that is required for the RNA and DNA polymerase enzymes involved in normal cellular growth and replication; thus, zinc is essential for epithelialization and fibroblast proliferation. Copper is a cofactor for cytochrome oxidase and superoxide dismutase. Iron is a cofactor in DNA replication and, along with vitamin C, in the hydroxylation of proline and lysine for collagen synthesis. Magnesium is a cofactor in the synthesis of protein and collagen. Deficiencies of these trace elements can lead to impaired collagen production and the retardation of healing [30].

Psychological Stress

Psychological stress can result in considerable impairment to wound healing. Stress disrupts inflammatory responses and cell-mediated immune functions at wound sites. It has been proposed that this disruption is primarily mediated through up-regulation of the hypothalamic-pituitary-adrenal and sympathetic-adrenal medullary axes [37]. Moreover, stress induces unhealthy behaviors, such as cigarette smoking, alcohol consumption, sleep disturbances and poor nutritional intake, all of which can aggravate the likelihood of impaired wound healing.

Obesity

Obese individuals often experience retarded wound healing and wound complications, such as wound infection, wound dehiscence and pressure ulcers [38]. These effects are likely explained in part by obesity-related local factors, including reduced vascularization of adipose tissues, skin folds that provide bacteria with moisture, friction caused by skin-on-skin contact, and increased tension at wound edges [38]. Additionally, adipose tissues have been reported to produce adipokines (leptin, adiponectin, resistin), cytokines (TNF-alpha, IL-1, IL-6, IL-8, IL-10), and chemokines (IL-8, monocyte chemoattractant protein-1 (MCP-1), interferon-gamma-indicible protein-10 (IP-10)). These bioactive substances cause alterations in systemic immunity and inflammatory responses [39, 40]. Obesity has also been associated with many diseases and conditions, such as atherosclerosis and type 2 diabetes, which increase the risk of wound impediment.

Alcohol and Smoking

Alcohol consumption and cigarette smoking are detrimental to wound healing. Acute ethanol exposure can impair the early inflammatory response by suppressing the release of pro-inflammatory cytokines and can diminish resistance to infection by inhibiting neutrophil migration and phagocytic functions [41]. In addition to its influence on the inflammatory phase of healing, ethanol disturbs angiogenesis, re-epithelialization, collagen production and the protease balance during the proliferative phase, with the greatest extent observed during wound angiogenesis [42]. Chronic alcohol exposure contributes to poor healing and to an increased risk of wound infection via different mechanisms.

In clinical practice, smokers display a delay in healing together with increased incidence of infection, decreased wound strength and wound rupture [43, 44]. These negative impacts of smoking have been shown to be attributed to some substances in cigarette smoke, such as nicotine, carbon monoxide, and hydrogen cyanide. Nicotine is a vasoconstrictor; thus, it reduces tissue blood flow and oxygenation [44]. Nicotine increases blood viscosity by increasing platelet adhesion and decreasing fibrinolysis. Nicotine also inhibits the proliferation of erythrocytes, macrophages and fibroblasts. Carbon monoxide reduces oxygen delivery to tissues by competing with oxygen to bind to hemoglobin in the circulation, while hydrogen cyanide interferes with cellular oxidative metabolism.

Medications

Any drugs that affect hemostasis, inflammatory responses and cell division can influence the healing cascade. For example, systemic corticosteroids, which are used as anti-inflammatory and immunosuppressive agents, not only inhibit wound repair by suppressing inflammatory responses, fibroblast proliferation and collagen synthesis, but they also increase susceptibility to infections [45, 46]. Conversely, the short-term use of topical corticosteroids has been reported to expedite wound healing when applied to chronic wound ulcers. Systemic non-steroidal anti-inflammatory drugs (NSAIDs) and chemotherapeutic agents have negative influences on healing because of their antiproliferative effects [45, 47].

Diabetes

Patients with diabetes are known to be vulnerable to impaired healing of acute cutaneous wounds and chronic diabetic foot ulcers. The pathophysiology of diabetes-induced impairment of healing is multiple and complex. The factors involved include the dysfunction of leukocytes, fibroblasts and keratinocytes [48], diminished host immunity [49], tissue hypoxia [50], impaired angiogenesis [51], increased protease levels [52], oxidative stress caused by hypoxia and hyperglycemia [53], increased formation of advanced glycation end-products (AGEs) [54], and neuropathy [55]. Mechanisms of diabetes-induced vascular complications leading to delayed wound healing are shown in Figure 2.

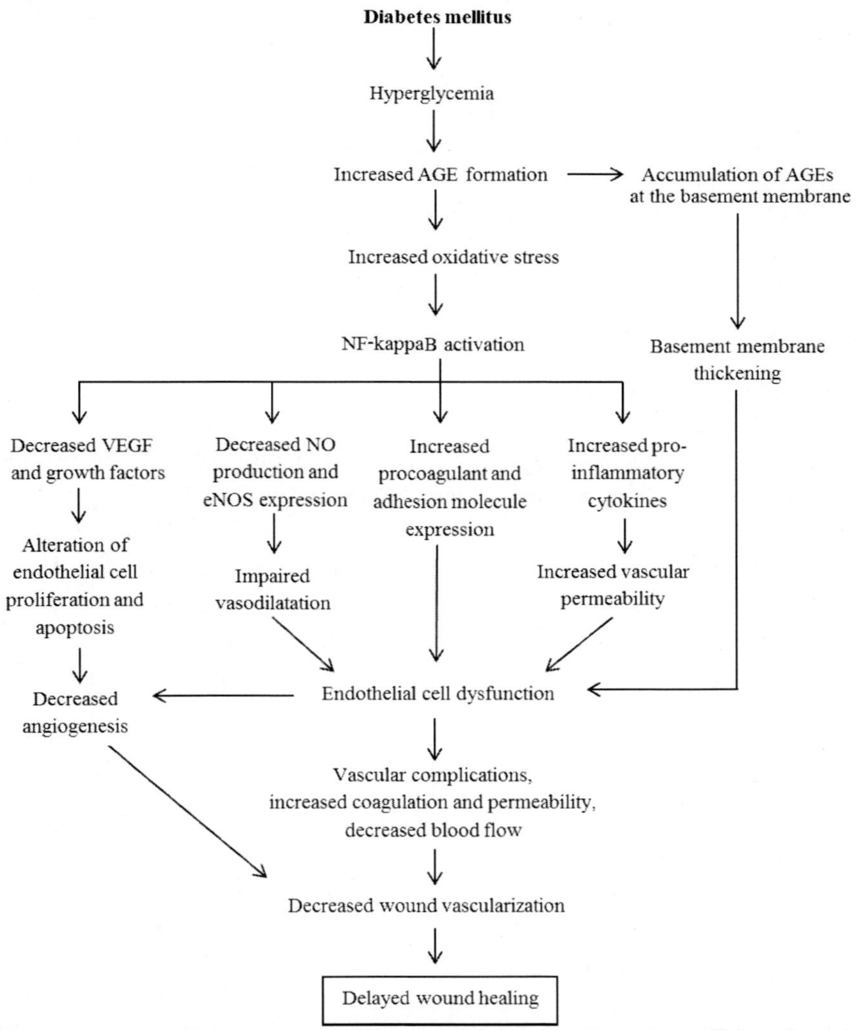

AGEs, advanced glycation end-products; eNOS, endothelial nitric oxide synthase; NF-kappaB, nuclear factor-kappaB; NO, nitric oxide; VEGF, vascular endothelial growth factor.

Figure 2. Mechanisms of diabetes-induced vascular complications leading to delayed wound healing.

Strategies for Wound Care Management

Wound care and management are principally aimed to accelerate healing with the maximum cosmetic and functional outcomes.

To achieve these aims, some associations, such as the Canadian Association for Wound Care (CAWC) and the Australian Wound Management Association (AWMA), have developed standards for wound management as tools to promote evidence-based best practices [56, 57].

According to the CAWC, strategies required for wound care and management include the following: 1) prevention strategies; 2) treatment strategies; 3) evaluation strategies; and 4) advanced treatment strategies (Table 2) [56]. Considering these guidelines and other related literature together, the aim and techniques of these strategies can be briefly described as follows.

Prevention Strategies

Prevention strategies include reducing or eliminating causative factors that delay healing while providing systemic support for healing, as well as supporting patient-centered concerns. Factors that influence the ability of wounds to heal, as mentioned previously, should be assessed and modified as optimally as possible. To address patient-centered concerns, the management of pain and quality of life should be assessed and supported. Additionally, patients and family members should be included in the management plan [56].

Treatment Strategies

Treatment strategies focus on infection prevention/control and on the provision of an optimal healing environment (wound moisture balance, optimum pH and temperature, protection against trauma). These strategies can be accomplished by the application of appropriate local wound care [56].

A wound assessment is performed to encompass all of the relevant aspects of the measurement parameters. These parameters, which can be easily memorized as the acronym "MEASURE", include the <u>m</u>easurement (length, width, depth and area), <u>e</u>xudate (amount, quality), <u>a</u>ppearance (wound bed appearance, tissue type and amount), <u>s</u>uffering (patient pain level), <u>u</u>ndermining (presence or absence), <u>r</u>e-evaluation (regular monitoring of all parameters) and edge (condition of the wound edge and surrounding skin) [56]. The presence and degree of wound infection must be determined. Wound infection can be treated with topically applied antimicrobials, whereas cellulitis that occurs around the wound should be treated with systemic, Gram-positive, bactericidal antibiotics [56, 57].

Wound cleansing must be performed to remove debris, devitalize tissues, and eliminate dressing residue and excessive or dry crusting exudate, using an aseptic or clean technique, according to the host system defense, the type of wound, and the healing environment. Sterile isotonic saline or water is the recommended cleansing product because it is non-toxic and has a neutral pH [58].

Debridement removes foreign debris and necrotic, contaminated tissues within the wound, thereby facilitating granulation tissue formation and allowing for wound closure. There are six debridement methods: surgical, sharp, enzymatic, autolytic, mechanical, and biological methods. Surgical debridement is indicated for extensive necrosis or heavily contaminated wounds, and it is a good choice for diabetic foot ulcers. Sharp debridement is less invasive than surgical methods. Enzymatic debridement involves the utilization of enzymatic preparations to degrade necrotic debris, and it is indicated for wounds with eschar and for friction-induced skin injuries. Autolytic debridement is performed with occlusive or semi-occlusive dressings, such as hydrocolloids, hydrogels and transparent films, which permit tissue autolysis via the body's own enzymes. This method is painless and thus indicated for patients with a low pain tolerance, such as in many cases of pediatric wounds, as well as cases of venous ulcers and traumatic ulcers with light eschar. Mechanical debridement is performed by physically removing debris with a wet-to-dry dressing, irrigation, pulsatile lavage or whirlpool therapy. In biological debridement, soft non-viable tissues are digested and ingested by maggots, the larvae of the greenbottle blowfly [59].

Wound dressings help to maintain continuous moisture in the wound bed, control the exudate and loosely obliterate the wound dead space. This process considers the proper type of dressing and the frequency of dressing changes. A dry, sterile dressing is appropriate for acute incisions that heal in response to primary intention, whereas a moist saline dressing works well for acute open wounds that have undergone secondary healing.

Exudative wounds require dressings with an absorptive capacity, such as alginate, hydrofiber and foam dressings. A low-adherence dressing is useful for acute minor wounds and for chronic wounds that have almost healed. Dressings that contain debriding agents are a good choice for necrotic wounds.

For dry necrotic wounds, hydrogel and hydrocolloid dressings are optimal for maintaining moisture while supporting autolytic debridement. Transparent film dressings, with no absorptive capacity and little hydrating ability are, suitable for clean, dry wounds [60].

Evaluation Strategies

The rate of wound healing should be evaluated, and if it is found to be suboptimal, the above strategies must be reassessed. For chronic wounds, a decrease in wound size by 20-40% within 2-4 weeks is indicative of healing [61].

Advanced Treatment Strategies

In the event that acute wounds develop complications, or healing does not progress despite the correction of other influential factors, active wound therapies, together with interprofessional care and a collaborative practice, could be required to improve outcomes.

Active wound therapies can involve the use of biological agents, skin grafts, and other adjunctive therapies, such as hyperbaric oxygen therapy, negative pressure therapy, electrical stimulation, ultrasound, laser light, hydrotherapy, vacuum-assisted wound closure, gene therapy, cytokines/growth factors, larvae, and dietary supplements.

Therefore, interdisciplinary and multidisciplinary health practitioners and team health workers must participate in the wound management team [56].

Experimental Approaches to Wound Healing

Wound research can be conducted both *in vivo* and *in vitro* to investigate different aspects of skin wound healing such as cellular and molecular mechanisms of acute wound healing, impaired healing conditions, and the efficacy of and mechanisms underlying new therapeutic modalities.

Table 2. Wound management strategies according to the Canadian Association of Wound Care

Strategies	Aims	Techniques
Prevention strategies	To reduce or eliminate the causative factors that delay healing To provide systemic support for healing	Assessing the patient's ability to heal, based on • Age • Nutritional status • Obesity • Alcohol and smoking • Vascularization • Oxygenation • Medication • Chronic diseases • Psychological stress and lack of sleep
		Managing comorbidities
	To address patient-centered concerns	Managing pain and quality of life
		Providing patient education and support
Treatment strategies	To provide a local wound environment that is optimal for healing • Debride necrotic tissue • Eliminate infection • Obliterate dead space • Absorb excess exudate • Maintain a moist environment • Protect against trauma and bacterial invasion • Provide thermal insulation	Applying appropriate local wound care • Wound assessment • Debridement • Wound cleansing • Infection prevention and control • Dressing
Evaluation strategies	To re-evaluate the progression of healing	Assessing and evaluating the rate of wound healing
Advanced treatment strategies	To improve treatment outcomes in the event of delayed healing	Using active wound therapies • Biological agents • Skin grafts • Adjunctive therapies (negative pressure therapy, hyperbaric oxygen therapy, electrical modalities, gene therapy, PDGF and vacuum-assisted wound closure)
		Employing interprofessional care and collaborative practices

PDGF, platelet-derived growth factor.

To date, an understanding of the major wound healing processes has been extensively established through decades of study. Current trends and future research are directed toward the development of effective therapies for wound healing problems and the optimization of normal healing processes.

This section provides a summary of the currently available *in vivo* and *in vitro* models of wound healing.

In Vivo Models of Wound Healing

Information regarding the nature of the wound healing process can be obtained using an *in vivo* model. *In vivo* studies in humans, however, are somewhat limited due to ethical issues, as well as variability in standards of clinical care, genetics and the environment. Therefore, animal models are usually employed in place of human subjects because of their advantages in terms of availability, reproducibility, cost effectiveness and standardization. Nevertheless, animal-based models do not perfectly represent the situation in humans because there are dissimilarities in skin structure, physiology, and immune response between humans and animals. The most ideal animal model for wound healing studies appears to be a porcine model, given that pigs and humans share very similar skin characteristics, such as tight skin adherence [62, 63]. However, rodents, such as rats and mice, despite having loose skin in which wound contraction is the main healing mechanism [64], are more widely used in wound-healing research because they are readily available, small in size, and inexpensive. Researchers have attempted to minimize the deviated pattern of wound healing in rodents compared to humans by utilizing wound splinting, which allows for re-epithelialization and granulation tissue formation [65, 66]. In addition to rats and mice, rabbits, dogs, and swine have also been used as animal models to study wound healing [67-69].

In an effort to mimic pathological healing or non-healing chronic wounds in humans, several animal models of impaired healing have evolved. Diabetic mice or rats appear to be the most widely used among these models [63]. Genetically deficient non-obese diabetic (NOD) mice and diabetic rats/mice induced with streptozotocin (STZ) or alloxan, which destroy pancreatic beta-cells, have been used as models of type 1 diabetes [70, 71]. Leptin (ob/ob)- or leptin receptor (db/db)-deficient mice and Zucker diabetic fatty (ZDF) rats have been used as research models of obesity and type 2 diabetes [72-74].

Modeling of aging involves the use of aged or ovariectomized rats/mice to mirror the human degenerative conditions that occur during aging and postmenopausal states [75, 76].

A skin flap model, which produces compromised cutaneous circulation with subsequent tissue necrosis and delayed wound repair, is an approach to healing impairment caused by tissue hypoxia [77]. Another model that has been exploited to imitate pressure sores in humans is the pressure model, which functions by creating tissue compression through the application of magnets onto the skin and a steel plate beneath the wound bed [78].

Four *in vivo* animal models are commonly utilized for wounding, including incision, excision, burn, and dead space wound models. Each model provides information regarding different aspects of wound healing; therefore, all of the models have benefits and limitations. As a general rule for the conducting of animal experimentation, general anesthesia is necessary prior to and during the process of wound creation. The skin must be shaved, depilated and disinfected prior to wounding. The wounds are typically made on the back of the animals so that they are protected against licking, biting or scratching by the animals. An overview of wound creation methods, an evaluation of wound healing processes, and the benefits/limitations of each wound model are provided below.

Incision Wound Model

An incision wound can be created along a paravertebral area through the entire thickness of the skin using a sharp blade or scalpel, causing acute skin disruption and bleeding. After complete hemostasis is achieved by direct pressure, the wound is closed with interrupted sutures to initiate healing principally by epithelialization, known as primary union or primary intention. The treatment modality is then applied during the experimental period, which usually lasts approximately 10 days [79, 80]. The sutures are removed on day 8 post-wounding, and the tissue is isolated from the healed wound for the determination of tensile strength (as indicated by the force required to break the wound) on day 10. Other studied parameters include the wound surface microbial load, collagen and protein contents, cutaneous blood flow, epidermal thickness, histology, immunohistochemistry, and *in situ* hybridization [64]. However, this type of wound is usually conducive to a limited healing area, making it a poor target for the evaluation of biochemistry and histology.

Excision Wound Model

The creation of an excisional wound involves the use of a surgical device, such as a sharp blade, scissors, a scalpel, biopsy punches or a dermatome, to remove the skin at the depth of the epidermis and upper dermis for a partial-thickness (or split-thickness) wound or both the epidermis and dermis to the fascia or subcutaneous tissue for a full-thickness wound [64, 81]. The wounds can be left open or covered with a dressing. As mentioned in the previous section, re-epithelialization originates from the wound margin and epidermal appendages, particularly the hair follicles. Thus, there is a high rate of re-epithelialization in the partial-thickness model, in which the bases of the hair follicles remain intact.

Consequently, hairless strains are more suitable for this model than other domestic animals that typically have high hair density [81]. The partial-thickness excisional wound model is useful for evaluating re-epithelialization rates, using either planimetric methods or histomorphometric analysis of serial sections [81]. Planimetry is the measurement of the wound surface area, which can be accurately performed by tracing the wound perimeter on a transparent sheet or on digital photographs. The analysis of a series of histological images is another method that is used to track changes in epithelialization over time.

For a full-thickness wound, healing occurs by contraction, re-epithelialization, and the formation of new tissue. Thus, this model allows for investigations into all aspects of healing. The size of the wound is measured to determine the period of epithelialization (the number of days required for full epithelialization without any residual raw wound) and the rate of wound contraction. Wound tissues can be harvested for histological, as well as molecular and cellular biological, assays, to evaluate granulation tissue formation, connective tissue organization, collagen or proteoglycan content, inflammation, angiogenesis, chemotaxis, and cell signaling cascades [81-83].

Dead Space Wound Model

In the dead space wound model, a chamber or sponge, made of porous, relatively inert, non-biodegradable materials, such as polyvinyl alcohol sponges, a Hunt-Schilling chamber, polytetrafluoroethylene tubing or sterile cotton pellets, is implanted subcutaneously into the groin or axilla to create an artificial tissue space, into which interstitial fluid diffuses [64]. This process activates fibrin clot formation and granulation tissue within the implant. Scar maturation can occur, and several layers of collagen fibers are usually deposited around the implant, giving rise to a connective tissue capsule.

The implant is then removed, and the granulation tissues are excised at approximately day 10 after wound infliction for further biochemical and histopathological assessments, such as collagen content, DNA content, breaking strength, and tissue organization [82]. The wound fluid that accumulates in the space during the early post-wounding period (days 3 to 5) can also be aspirated for biochemical analyses of metabolites, cytokines, growth factors, and non-adherent cells [81]. To examine the actions of therapeutic agents in wound repair, test agents can be injected or implanted into the chamber, in addition to oral administration [81]. Although this model allows for the study of the process of connective tissue formation, it should be noted that some limitations still exist.

The implant can interfere with normal scar maturation and can cause foreign body reactions. Additionally, the epithelialization component of healing is lacking in this wound model [81].

Burn Wound Model

Several animal models for thermal burns of varying degrees have been developed by the use of scalding or using a heated conductive device that is placed onto the shaved skin and has a controlled temperature, area, and duration of exposure. For example, to create a partial-thickness or second-degree burn, a hot plate (3.5 × 4.6 cm), at a temperature of 75°C, is placed on the dorsal skin of Wistar rats for 10 seconds [84]. Interestingly, using an identical temperature and infliction time, the 75°C, 10-second guinea pig scald burn was found to produce full-thickness skin loss, particularly in cases in which the blister is ruptured [85]. A round aluminum stamp (4 cm in diameter, 85 g) heated to 80°C and applied for 14 seconds also yields a partial-thickness burn in the dorsal skin of rabbits [86]. A deep partial-thickness burn, in which the damage extends to the deep dermis, is obtained with an aluminum bar weighing 51 g (10 mm in diameter), which is preheated to 100°C/10 min and is placed on the skin of Wistar rats for 15 seconds [87]. The application of a copper plate heated to 200°C to the skin of Wistar rats for 9 seconds results in full-thickness or third-degree burns without central re-epithelialization, while temperatures of 100°C and 150°C produce partial-thickness burns, with only burning at 100°C resulting in central re-epithelialization [88].

According to a systematic review of experimental models for burns in rats (from 2008 to January 2011), the majority of the burns studied were third degree burns produced using hot water as the main method. It was concluded that the studies were not very reproducible [89].

Therefore, it is important to note that, following wound infliction using any of these experimental burn models, the depth and degree of the burn lesions must be verified histologically.

Similar to the aforementioned wound models, the assessment of burn wound healing, including monitoring of the healing rate, as well as biochemical and histopathological evaluations, is performed in research. Because burn injury always produces considerable vascular damage and acute inflammatory responses, other aspects of wound healing to be investigated have also focused on the microcirculation, vascular-related growth factors (such as VEGF and FGF; see the previous section), and pro-inflammatory cytokines and related mediators [84, 90].

Burn models are amenable to the evaluation of novel therapeutics, such as volume therapy, nutrition and rehabilitation, skin grafting, gene therapy, drug therapy and topical agents, and herbal medicine [91].

An interesting technique that is used for the study of wound microcirculation is the incorporation of a dorsal skinfold chamber preparation and intravital microscopy [92]. The chamber frames are implanted into the dorsal skin flap, of which the layers encompassed in the observation window of the chamber are the epidermis, subcutaneous tissue and striated muscle. Dermal microvascular changes are then studied using intravital fluorescence microscopy, with intravenously injected fluorescein isothiocyanate (FITC)-labeled dextran and acridine orange as fluorescent markers to provide contrast enhancement for the visualization of plasma and leukocytes, respectively. This technique allows for quantitative studies of the hemodynamic and morphologic microvasculature, including the microvessel diameter and red blood cell velocity in arterioles (16 to 50 microns in diameter), capillaries (4 to 9 microns in diameter), and post-capillary venules (19 to 60 microns in diameter), leukocyte-endothelium interactions (as characterized by leukocyte adhesion to the endothelium of postcapillary venules for at least 30 seconds), functional capillary density and intercapillary distance, and endothelial cell integrity [92].

In Vitro Models of Wound Healing

To reduce the use of live animals and to avoid uncontrolled systemic variables within the body, *in vitro* systems have been developed as alternatives to animal model systems. One of the most readily available and widely used *in vitro* techniques is the simple cell assay [63], such as the fibroblast cell assay used to determine wound healing activity in the context of fibroblast proliferation, based on neutral red uptake [93]. An *in vitro* model that can be used for the study of angiogenesis is the chorioallantoic membrane model, using 9-day-old embryonated chicken eggs from which the albumin is removed on day 4 after fertilization [94]. A more intricate system is a "three-dimensional skin equivalent" model, using keratinocytes cultured on a fibroblast layer within a collagen gel [95]. In an attempt to mirror the *in vivo* situation, another model, known as the *ex vivo* skin explant system, has been developed [96]. Such models utilize whole excised human skin obtained from skin biopsies or during surgical procedures, such as breast reduction operations and cosmetic procedures.

Wounds (incisional and burn wounds) with a standardized area and depth are created in the *ex vivo* skin samples, which are then incubated *in vitro*.

The viability of the cells from the wounds is maintained for 14 days [97, 98] or even up to 21 days [99] of the incubation (also called culture) period, during which wound re-epithelialization, as well as fibroblast migration and proliferation, can be assessed using histological and immunohistochemical analyses.

The *in vitro* models are useful for the study of individual healing processes, such as cell migration and re-epithelialization, as well as the effects of the tested agents and treatments on the wound healing process. However, the *in vitro* systems still have some limitations, including the lack of an *in vivo* wound environment, an inability to determine the systemic or adverse effects of the treatments applied, and a short-lived viability that enables the study of only the early phases of wound healing [63].

Part II: Herbal Medicine for Cutaneous Wounds

Currently, herbal medicine has gained increasing interest in wound care. Considering its popularity, a number of investigations into the therapeutic roles of medicinal plants in wound management have been conducted in human and animal models. Among the well-recognized and most studied medicinal plants are *Aloe vera*, *Centella asiatica* and *Curcuma longa.*

The following sections provide information on these herbal plants with regard to botany, chemical constituents, traditional use, and related evidence regarding their efficacy and therapeutic properties in animal and human studies. The mechanisms underlying how these three medicinal plants exert beneficial effects on wound healing are discussed in the context of their roles in each key component of the healing process.

Important components for optimal wound healing are generally considered to include the following: appropriate inflammation; mesenchymal cell differentiation; proliferation; migration to the wound site; legitimate angiogenesis; expeditious re-epithelialization; and proper synthesis and remodeling of collagen to provide healed tissue strength [100].

Aloe Vera and Its Mechanisms in Wound Healing

Aloe vera is a plant that belongs to the Liliacea (Asphodelaceae) family, which comprises approximately 360 species. The scientific name is *Aloe vera* (Linn.) Burm. f., and it is also known as *Aloe barbadensis* Miller, *Aloe indica* Royle, *Aloe perfoliata* L. var. *vera*, and *Aloe vulgaris* Lam. *Aloe vera* is a short-stemmed perennial succulent that grows mainly in most of the tropics and in hot and dry climates in regions of Africa, Asia, Europe and the Americas [101]. It has fleshy, triangle-shaped leaves with a sharp apex and spiny edges. The outermost layer of the leaf has a thick cuticle. The middle layer consists of pericyclic cells, which contain the bitter yellow latex known as aloe juice. The innermost part of the leaf is the colorless pulp, which consists of mucilaginous cells containing the thick, glue-like gel called *Aloe vera* gel [102].

Chemical studies have revealed that the latex portion, or aloe juice, contains anthraquinone derivatives and their glycosides, such as barbaloin, isobarbaloin, anthranol, aloe emodin, emodin, aloetic acid, and ester of cinnamic acids, among others. The aloe gel within the leaf pulp consists of 99.5% water and 0.5% solid components. The vast majority of substances present in the solid component are mixed polysaccharides (97%), with acemannan as the primary polysaccharide. These polysaccharides consist of several monosaccharides (predominantly mannose 6-phosphate).

The remaining constituents of the solid component include proteins, lipids, amino acids, vitamins, enzymes, and inorganic and organic compounds [103]. It should be noted that the chemical constituents of aloe gel vary with the planting location and the age of the plant [103, 104].

Aloe vera has long been used for many indications, since the time of the Roman Empire or perhaps as long before that time as in ancient Egypt. To date, it is a popular herb that is used to treat wounds as part of traditional herbal medicine in many countries, such as China, India, Japan, the West Indies and South Africa [101, 105]. In Thailand, the Ministry of Public Health has also incorporated *Aloe vera* into the Thai Fundamental Public Health Drug List for the treatment of burn wounds [106]. The traditional use of *Aloe vera* for the treatment of wounds involves the application of the mucilaginous gel from the fresh leaf to burned or inflamed skin.

Research over several decades has demonstrated the beneficial effects of *Aloe vera* during various stages of the wound healing process. In 2004, a review by Somboonwong and Duansak indicated that the efficacy of topical *Aloe vera* gel in thermal burn therapy was mediated through different actions, including anti-inflammation, antimicrobials, wound healing promotion, and biological/immunological modulation [107]. Currently, much more evidence has provided the cellular and molecular details of the mechanisms of action underlying its suppression of wound inflammation, stimulation of angiogenesis, re-epithelialization, and enhancement of matrix formation and remodeling.

Role of *Aloe Vera* in the Suppression of Wound Inflammation

It is known that appropriate inflammation, which occurs in a consecutive, self-limited, controlled manner, is required for adequate wound healing. In addition, a decreased inflammatory response helps to relieve pain, heat, redness and swelling. Furthermore, an excessive or prolonged inflammatory response can lead to chronic healing. It is also noteworthy that inhibition of COX-2-mediated inflammation and the resultant reduction in PGE2 have been reported to reduce scar generation, without any effects on the re-epithelialization or tensile strength of the wound, as evident in scarless, complete fetal wound healing without inflammation [108].

Aloe vera has been shown to be effective in suppressing wound inflammation. According to Fulton, dressing wounds with aloe gel after facial dermabrasion in acne patients shortened the healing time and resulted in the reduction of edema and vasoconstriction at the wound site between 24 and 48 hours [109].

Aloe vera can attenuate cutaneous microvascular changes during the inflammatory phase of a burn wound [84, 90, 110, 111]. These inhibitory effects of *Aloe vera* were demonstrated *in vivo* by Somboonwong et al., using intravital fluorescent microscopic monitoring. After inflicting second-degree burn wounds in rats, prominent vasodilation of subcutaneous arterioles and capillary tortuousity were observed on day 7 post-burn, followed by arteriolar constriction on day 14. Increased permeability of postcapillary venules, sustained adherence of leukocytes on postcapillary venules, and transmigration of leukocytes into the interstitium were observed at both time points. Therefore, it was clearly demonstrated that second-degree burns produced an acute inflammatory response, as evidenced by endothelial and microvascular injury and by microvascular morphological changes. When treated with topical lyophilized aloe gel, these alterations were ameliorated, and the wounds healed significantly more rapidly than untreated wounds or those treated with normal saline, a solution that is used practically for wound dressing [84].

A subsequent study conducted by Duansak et al., using a similar burn model and a microcirculation study technique to examine the effects of *Aloe vera* on leukocyte-endothelial interactions and serum levels of the inflammatory cytokines TNF-alpha and IL-6. Notably, *Aloe vera* could decrease the degree of leukocyte adhesion and the levels of these cytokines [90].

The inhibition by *Aloe vera* of vascular changes following a burn injury was further confirmed by Lv et al., using a deep partial-thickness burn wound model in rats [110]. They found that topical treatment with either raw aloe polysaccharide or aloe gel decreased nitric oxide content, optimized the nitric oxide-to-endothelin ratio, reduced the vascular inflammatory reaction and diminished permeability and edema in wound tissues, compared to sulfadiazine pyridine silver cream and normal saline [110].

Figure 3 depicts the mechanisms of action underlying the effects of *Aloe vera* on the suppression of wound inflammation, involving inhibition of the activities of the mediators and cytokines released during the inflammatory phase of wound healing, as described below.

Antithromboxane/Antiprostaglandin Activities

A body of evidence has shown that *Aloe vera* blocks prostaglandin and thromboxane synthesis, which supports the inhibitory activity of *Aloe vera* in arachidonic acid metabolism via the cyclooxygenase (COX) pathway. An *in vitro* study conducted by Penneys showed that unspecified substances in aloe gel inhibited the oxidation of arachidonic acid, which is the substrate required for the synthesis of thromboxanes and prostaglandins [112]. *In vivo*, Heggers et al. demonstrated that *Aloe vera* could inhibit localized TXA2 production and thereby reduce vasoconstriction, which in turn protected wounded tissue against a progressive decrease in blood supply and increased tissue survival in patients with burns, frostbite, electrical injuries, distal dying flaps, or intra-arterial drug abuse [113]. Other arachidonic acid metabolites generated after burn injuries, such as TXB2 and prostaglandin F_2-alpha (PGF2-alpha), which cause dermal ischemia, were also reduced by aloe, as stated by Robson et al. [114]. Similarly, *Aloe vera* was able to reduce the vasoconstriction that occurred 14 days after burning, as previously mentioned in the study reported by Somboonwong et al. [84]. The unpublished data obtained from our research group using laser Doppler flowmetry corroborated the positive effects of aloe on the tissue perfusion of burn wounds at all of the monitored time points (days 3, 7 and 14 post-burn).

There are several active ingredients in aloe gel that exert antithromboxane and antiprostaglandin activities. Aloe gel contains steroids [115], which block prostaglandin synthesis by inhibiting phospholipase A2, thus reducing arachidonic acid release from phospholipids. *Aloe vera* sterols (a subgroup of steroids), including lupeol, campesterol, and beta-sitosterol, exhibit anti-inflammatory activities, as evidenced by a reduction in croton oil-induced ear swelling, with lupeol demonstrating the greatest efficacy in reducing inflammation (by 37.0%) [116]. In addition, lectin aloctin A, which is a glycoprotein that is isolated from aloe gel, was found to inhibit carrageenan-induced edema in rats [117] and to modulate PGE2 production *in vitro* [118]. *Aloe vera* also provides salicylic acid, an aspirin-like substance, which is known to disrupt COX enzyme activity [119]. Additionally, aloesin derivatives, including p-coumaroylaloesin and feruloylaloesin, were shown to have inhibitory effects on COX-2 and TXA2 synthase [120].

It should be noted that, despite the presence of substances that inhibit the production of prostaglandin and thromboxane, *Aloe vera* extracts have also been found to contain COX enzyme, which converts arachidonic acids into different prostanoids. This conversion, in turn counteracts, the enzyme's own antithromboxane and antiprostaglandin activities [121].

Antileukotriene Activity

Another family of arachidonic acid metabolites that are synthesized by lipoxygenase (LOX) enzyme is the leukotrienes, which cause vasoconstriction, increased microvascular permeability and leukocyte adhesion. The aforementioned studies by Somboonwong et al. and Duansak et al., showing reductions of postcapillary venular permeability and leukocyte adherence in aloe-treated burn wounds, indicated a possible role for *Aloe vera* in the inhibition of the LOX pathway of arachidonic acid metabolism [84, 90]. However, direct evidence for the antileukotriene activity of *Aloe vera* has been documented in allergic reactions such as asthma, in which alprogen, a glycoprotein component that is purified from aloe, inhibits leukotriene release by inhibiting mass 1,2-diacylglycerol formation and phospholipase activity during the activation of guinea pig lung mast cells [122].

Antibradykinin Activity

Another activity that contributes to the anti-inflammatory effects of *Aloe vera* is the inhibition of bradykinin activity. *Aloe vera* contains antibradykinin enzymes, such as bradykininase [123] and carboxypeptidase [124], which hydrolyze bradykinin and angiotensin I to be converted into angiotensin II.

The activity of bradykininase and carboxypeptidase extracted from aloe subsequently results in the suppression of vasodilatation and pain at the site of acute inflammation, as reported by Rubel [125] and by Klein and Penneys [102], respectively. Aloe glycoprotein has also been reported to be an active antibradykinin constituent due to the presence of carboxypeptidase N- and P-like enzymes [126].

Antihistamine Activity

Aloe vera consists of magnesium lactate, barbaloin and aloctin, which possess antihistamine activity that aids in reducing vasodilatation, inflammation, and pruritus. It has been demonstrated that magnesium lactate prevents the conversion of histidine into histamine in mast cells by inhibiting histidine decarboxylase [127], whereas barbaloin and aloctin prevent histamine release from mast cells [128].

Inhibition of Pro-Inflammatory Cytokine and Enzyme Activity

As mentioned previously, *Aloe vera* can prevent an increase in circulating levels of inflammatory cytokines, such as TNF-alpha and IL-6, as well as endothelium-leukocyte interactions, following burn injury [90]. During the early burn phase, at 0-72 hours, cells at the injury site, mainly tissue macrophages, are triggered to release pro-inflammatory or first-wave cytokines, such as TNF-alpha and IL-1, which, concomitantly with other soluble mediators, such as histamine, induce adhesive molecule expression on endothelial cells and stimulate COX activity. This phenomenon is followed by a cascade release of second-wave cytokines, such as IL-6 and IL-8, which can give rise to local and systemic inflammation or eventually multiple organ failure. The interactions among these cytokines are complex. For example,

TNF-alpha mediates inflammatory action and stimulates fibroblasts and angiogenesis while also participating in the development of multiple organ failure after burn injuries [129, 130]. There is evidence that increased circulating TNF-alpha levels indicate a poor prognosis for burns [131]. Inversely, IL-6 inhibits TNF-alpha synthesis and decreases the severity of inflammation during the early phases of burn injuries [132]. Given the effects of *Aloe vera* on anti-inflammatory cytokine activity and epidermal cell growth promotion, Duansak et al. reported that *Aloe vera* might expedite the turnover rate of these inflammatory cytokines that cause wound healing processes to resolve rapidly [90].

A member of the gelatinase family of MMPs, MMP-9, which is known to have many pro-inflammatory actions in wound healing, is also downregulated by *Aloe vera.* An observation reported by Vijayalakshmi et al. suggested that the anti-inflammatory activity of *Aloe vera* is mediated by inhibition of the activity and production of MMP-9 in peripheral blood mononuclear cells [133].

Antioxidant Activity

There is a relationship between anti-inflammatory activity and radical scavenging capacity. Although low levels of reactive oxygen species are required for optimal wound healing, exaggerated oxidative stress results in impaired wound healing.

Free radicals that are generated during the inflammatory process enhance the production of the pro-inflammatory cytokines TNF-alpha, IL-1 and IL-8 by activating nuclear factor-kappa-B (NF-κB). Evidence from *in vitro* and *in vivo* animal studies has suggested that antioxidants reduce NF-κB activation and thereby prevent the up-regulation of pro-inflammatory cytokines [134, 135]. Antioxidant therapy has been shown to protect the microcirculation and to reduce tissue lipid peroxidation in burn-mediated trauma [136].

In vitro studies have identified antioxidant components of *Aloe vera,* including aloesin derivatives (isorabaichromone, feruloylaloesin, and p-coumaroylaloesin), polysaccharides, flavonoids, polyphenols, indoles, and alkaloids [137-139]. However, direct documentation of the effects of *Aloe vera* on oxidative stress in the wound is not available.

Other Activities

In addition to the activities described above, *Aloe vera* gel also exerts anti-inflammatory actions via other activities, some of which have not yet been defined. For example, certain amino acids, vitamins, and mannose present in

Aloe vera have strong anti-inflammatory effects because they are capable of normalizing acute vascular responses [119, 140].

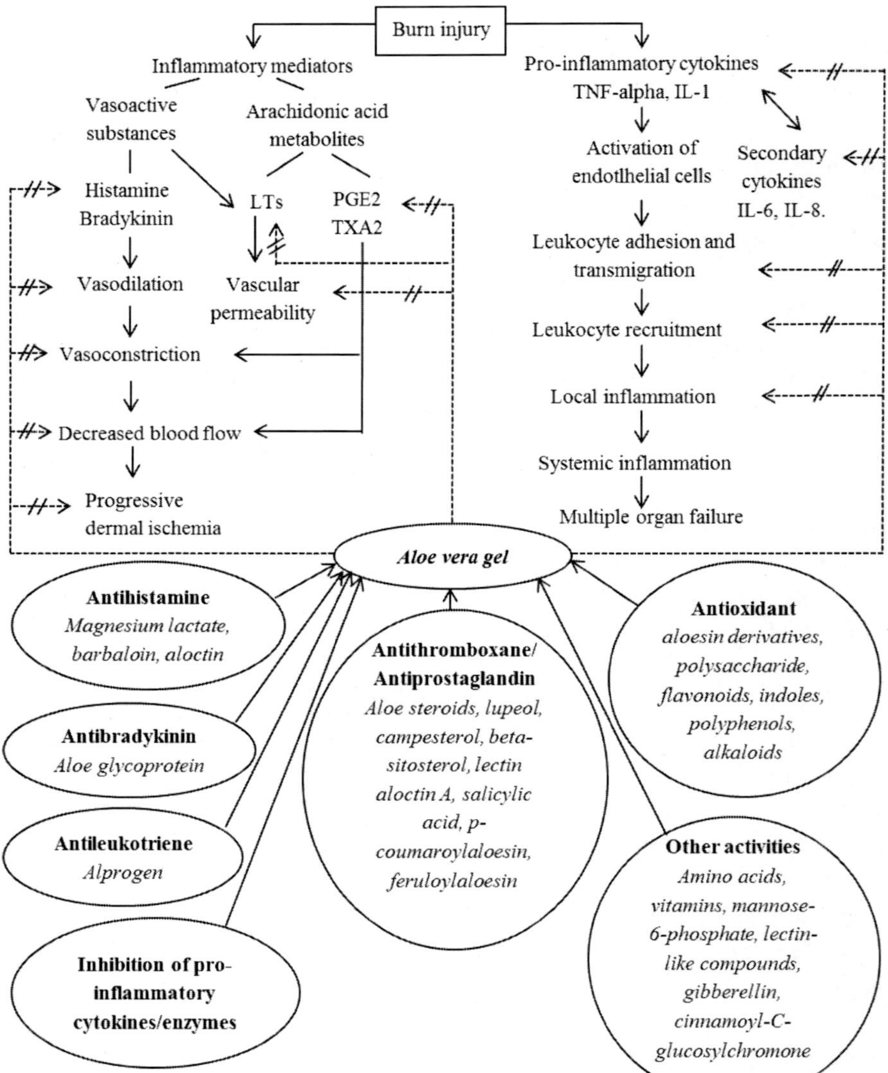

IL-6, interleukin-6; IL-8, interleukin-8; LTs, leukotrienes; PGE2, prostaglandin E2; TNF-alpha, tumor necrosis factor-alpha; TXA2, thromboxane A2.

Figure 3. Mechanisms of *Aloe vera* gel and its components (in italic text) in the suppression of wound inflammation.

It has been suggested that certain amino acids and vitamins synergistically trigger the activities of the enzymes and polysaccharides that are required for anti-inflammatory activities [141]. Mannose-6-phosphate might act by inhibiting the degradation of the vascular basement membrane ECM, thus preventing leukocyte extravasation to the site of injury.

The mechanism underlying the anti-inflammatory effect of mannose-6-phosphate is presumably inhibition of the lysosomal enzyme-mannose phosphate receptor interaction [142]. Aloe preparations also contain lectin-like compounds, gibberellin, and cinnamoyl-C-glucosylchromone, which are capable of reducing inflammation [143-145].

Role of *Aloe Vera* in Wound Angiogenesis

Angiogenesis plays a vital role in accelerating wound repair because this process of new capillary vessel formation provides microvascular perfusion that brings nutrients and oxygen to the wounded area. A reduction in angiogenesis engenders wound healing challenges, such as diabetic foot ulceration [146]. In the wounds of diabetic animals, angiogenic growth factors, such as FGF-2, VEGF and PDGF, have also been reported to be depleted [147-149]. Moreover, topical application of VEGF has been shown to promote the healing of nondiabetic ischemic wounds [150] and diabetic wounds [151] via increases in angiogenesis. Currently, the stimulation of angiogenesis with several interventions has been integrated into chronic wound treatments [152].

Aloe vera gel has been shown to possess angiogenic properties. Davis et al. demonstrated that, after wound infliction on the backs of mice using a punch biopsy, topical and oral *Aloe vera* effectively decreased wound diameters, and increased vascularization was noted around the wounded area upon histological examination [153]. According to Heggers et al., a restoration of vascularity was also observed after aloe gel was topically applied to burn wounds induced in guinea pigs [154]. The number of blood vessel sections within sutured incision wounds created in rats also increased with topical *Aloe vera* gel beginning on day 4 post-wounding, compared with thyroid hormone cream, silver sulfadiazine cream and vehicle [155]. In addition to the benefits to nondiabetic wounds, oral administration of *Aloe vera* was shown to increase angiogenesis in delayed healing wounds in the two studies reported by Atiba et al. [156, 157]. In the first example in full-thickness open wounds in type 2 diabetic rats, aloe worked via the activation of VEGF and transforming growth factor (TGF)-beta 1 expression [156]. In another study of radiation-exposed rats, aloe stimulated the production of TGF-beta and bFGF [157].

The ability of *Aloe vera* to promote angiogenesis has been accounted for by some of its active components. Lee et al. showed that low-molecular-weight substances present in the methanol-soluble fraction of dichloromethane extracts of lyophilized *Aloe vera* gel augmented angiogenesis in a chick embryo chorioallantoic membrane (CAM) assay [158]. A subsequent study by the same research group showed that the most active fraction (F3) of the dichloromethane extract of aloe gel increased the proliferation of calf pulmonary artery endothelial cells and the differentiation of these cells into capillary-like tubes. This F3 fraction also enhanced the expression of urokinase-type plasminogen activator (u-PA), MMP-2, and membrane-type MMP (MT-MMP), all of which are proteolytic enzymes that are used in ECM degradation to establish an environment for the process of capillary sprouting during angiogenesis [159].

Beta-sitosterol is a low-molecular-weight compound that is an active angiogenic factor obtained from *Aloe vera* gel. As reported by Moon et al., beta-sitosterol has potent angiogenic activity in CAM assay and promotes the formation of new blood vessels in mouse Matrigel plug assay. These effects were partly due to the stimulation of endothelial cell migration, as evidenced by an increase in the motility of human umbilical vein endothelial cells in wound migration assay [160]. Choi et al. also confirmed the angiogenic effects of beta-sitosterol isolated from *Aloe vera* gel on the damaged blood vessels of Mongolian gerbil brains using ischemia/reperfusion.

Moreover, they demonstrated an increase in the expression levels of proteins involved in angiogenesis, such as VEGF, VEGF-R2 or fetal liver kinase-1 (Flk-1), von Willebrand factor (a marker for blood endothelial cells), and blood vessel matrix laminin (a principal component of the basement membranes that underlie the endothelium) [161].

In addition, acemannan, a major polysaccharide of *Aloe vera* gel, has been reported to affect angiogenesis positively. In the study reported by Jettanacheawchankit et al. using a [(3)H]-thymidine incorporation assay and ELISA, acemannan accelerated oral wound healing in rats by inducing fibroblast proliferation and activating the expression of VEGF, keratinocyte growth factor-1 (KGF-1), and type I collagen [162].

Considering all of the above findings, it can be concluded that *Aloe vera* gel and its isolated constituents, such as the fraction containing low-molecular-weight substances, beta-sitosterol and acemannan, appear to play positive roles in the stimulation of wound angiogenesis. As illustrated in Figure 4, *Aloe vera* appears to influence every step in the wound angiogenic process. The angiogenic action of *Aloe vera* can be explained mainly by two mechanisms: an increase in the expression levels of key angiogenic growth factors, such as VEGF and FGF-2; and up--regulation of the protease enzymes involved in ECM degradation.

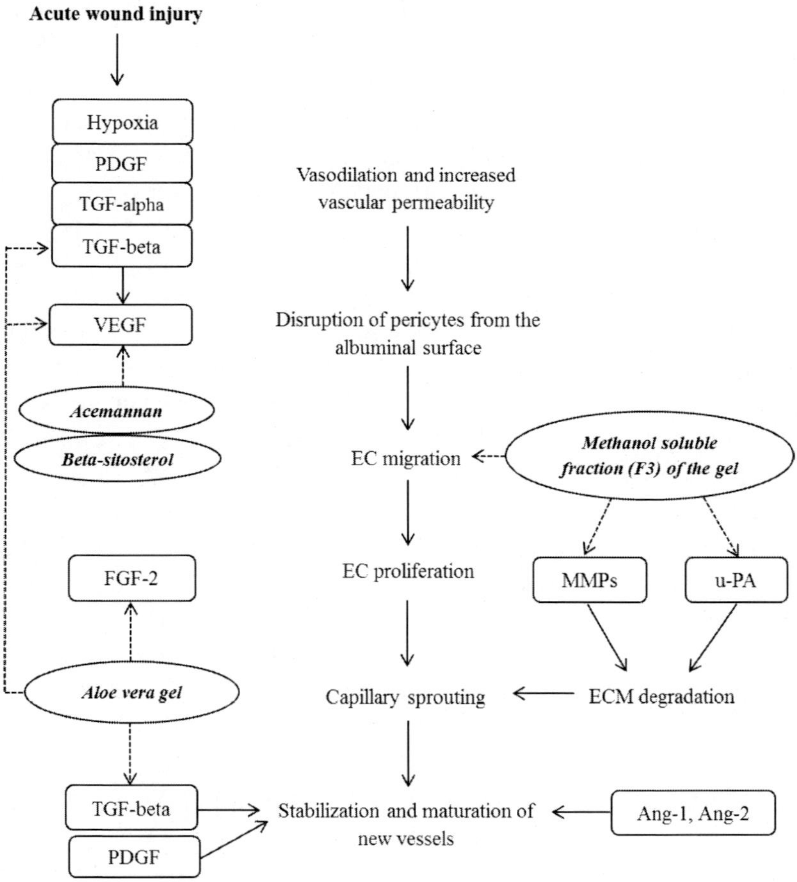

Ang-1, Ang-2, angiogenins 1 and 2; EC, endothelial cell; FGF-2, fibroblast growth factor-2 or basic fibroblast growth factor; MMPs, matrix metalloproteinases; PDGF, platelet-derived growth factor; TGF-beta, transforming growth factor-beta; u-PA, urokinase-type plasminogen activator; VEGF, vascular endothelial growth factor.

Figure 4. Mechanisms of *Aloe vera* gel and its components (in bold, italic text) in the stimulation of wound angiogenesis via activation of the expression of growth factors and proteolytic enzymes.

Role of *Aloe Vera* in Wound Re-Epithelialization

Wound closure requires effective re-epithelialization, in addition to wound contraction. Re-epithelialization occurs based on a combination of keratinocyte proliferation, migration, and differentiation.

Two mechanisms are independently involved in this process: the passive displacement of the superficial layers near the wound edge; and the migration of keratinocytes over one another [163]. Several experimental *in vivo* studies have provided results that support the positive effects of *Aloe vera* gel on the epithelialization of full-thickness excisional [157, 164], incisional [155], and burn wounds [165, 166]. A similar effect was also observed in burn patients, particularly those suffering from superficial and partial-thickness burns [167].

The mechanism of action of *Aloe vera* and its components in promoting wound epithelialization occurs via the activation of certain growth factors (Figure 5). According to Choi et al., a glycoprotein fraction of *Aloe vera,* namely G1G1M1DI2, which has a molecular weight of 5.5 kDa, stimulates epidermal proliferation in cell culture, concomitant with an increase in the expression of proliferation markers, including EGF receptor, fibronectin receptor, fibronectin, keratin 5/14 and keratin 1/10.

This fraction also accelerates the migration of human keratinocytes. The stimulating effects of this fraction on both cell proliferation and migration thus underlie the wound healing effects of *Aloe vera* [168].

Acemannan can stimulate the expression of KGF-1, which is a growth factor that regulates the migration and proliferation of keratinocytes [162]. In addition, *Aloe vera* extract has been reported to stimulate the expression of FGF-2, leading to increased keratinocyte proliferation [169].

Role of *Aloe Vera* in Fibroblast Proliferation, Matrix Formation, and Remodeling

Aloe vera has important attributes in the synthesis of glycosaminoglycan components in the provisional matrix and connective tissue matrix. A series of *in vivo* studies undertaken by Chithra et al. using a full-thickness wound rat model showed that *Aloe vera* increased the synthesis and turnover of glycosaminoglycans, particularly hyaluronic acid and dermatan sulfate, in the provisional matrix of the healing wound [170]. Furthermore, *Aloe vera* not only increased the collagen content of the granulation tissue formed within the wound, but it also affected the collagen characteristics by increasing crosslinking and enhancing type III collagen, as indicated by a reduction in the ratio of type I/type III collagen [171]. Additionally, *Aloe vera* promoted collagen turnover (collagen synthesis and its degradation) as well as collagen maturation, as indicated by the elevation of lysyl oxidase, which is involved in crosslinking newly synthesized collagen [172]. This research group also confirmed the beneficial effects of *Aloe vera* on fibroplasia and collagen synthesis and maturation in diabetic wound healing [173].

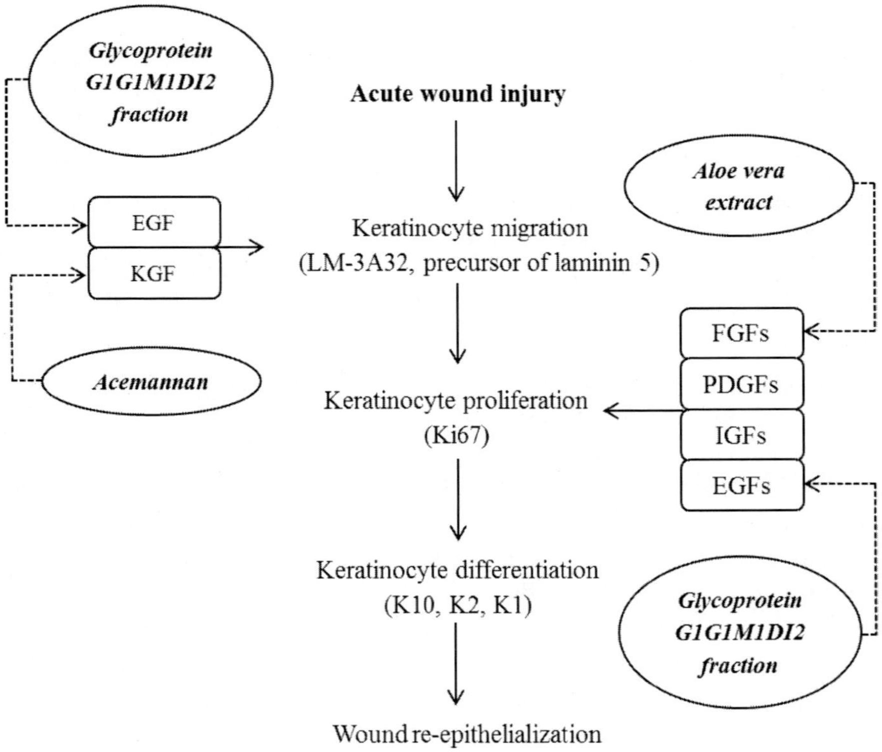

EGF, epithelial growth factor; FGFs, fibroblast growth factors; IGFs, insulin-like growth factors; KGF, keratinocyte growth factor; PDGFs, platelet-derived growth factors.

Figure 5. Mechanisms by which *Aloe vera* gel and its components (in bold, italic text) stimulate wound epithelialization via the activation of certain growth factors. The biomarkers of keratinocyte migration, proliferation, and differentiation in the re-epithelialization process are presented in brackets.

A very recent work of Oryan et al. has also validated the acceleration of cutaneous wound healing, modeling and remodeling in response to *Aloe vera* [174]. They reported that a 10-day topical application of *Aloe vera* (25 and 50 mg/mL) not only modulated inflammation but also increased wound contraction and epithelialization. The scar tissue was decreased in size with increased alignment and organization of the regenerated scar tissue. The treated wounds had a higher content of collagen and glycosaminoglycans, a greater maximum load, ultimate strength, and modulus of elasticity, compared to the saline controls [174].

Figure 6 reveals the mechanisms underlying *Aloe vera* gel and its components in extracellular matrix formation and remodeling via the stimulation of growth factors. *Aloe vera* has been shown to stimulate the proliferation of fibroblasts, which are the key cells in the production of extracellular matrix during the proliferative phase of the healing process. It has been found that *Aloe vera* increases the number of fibroblasts when it is topically applied on surgical incisions *in vivo* [155] This effect has been confirmed in a number of *in vitro* studies [162, 169, 175-177]. Abdullah et al. demonstrated an increase in gap junctional intercellular communication and proliferation of diabetic skin fibroblasts in cultures with *Aloe vera* extract, which was suggested to function by either binding to FGF-2 receptors or affecting the FGF-2 signaling pathway [175].

Aloe vera polysaccharide has been demonstrated to be the responsible constituent because it can induce fibroblast proliferation [176, 177] as well as hyaluronic acid and hydroxyproline production in human fibroblasts [177]. As previously mentioned in the study by Jettanacheawchankit et al., acemannan, which contains mannose-6-phosphate as a main sugar, increases type I collagen production and activates the expression of KGF-1, a growth factor that stimulates fibroblast proliferation [162]. It has also been reported that mannose-6-phosphate binds to the same receptor on fibroblasts as insulin-like growth factor II but at separate binding sites, possibly activating fibroblast proliferation [178, 179]. Additionally, Inpanya et al. have demonstrated that skin fibroblasts cultured on fibroin film composite with aloe gel extract exhibit an increase in attachment and proliferation along with enhanced bFGF expression by immunofluorescence. Furthermore, this aloe-containing fibroin film, when used to dress diabetic wounds, could expedite healing and restore the fibroblast distribution and the arrangement of collagen fibers in the wounds [169].

Other substances present in *Aloe vera* also have growth-promoting and wound healing activities. Not only mannose-6-phosphate but also gibberellin and auxins are also known plant-derived growth factors [178, 179]. Lectin-like compounds in leaf extracts promote the growth of normal human cells and enhance the healing of wounded cell monolayers in tissue culture [180]. A glycoprotein (Pg 21-2b fraction) isolated from *Aloe vera* gel augments human normal dermal cell proliferation [181].

Although *Aloe vera* appears to enhance fibroblast proliferation, an *in vitro* cell migration assay using cultured fibroblasts post-infliction revealed no direct effect of aloe on increasing the motility of fibroblasts [182].

One of the explanations for the stimulating effect of *Aloe vera* on collagen synthesis is simply the presence of glycine, proline, and lysine, which are the principal amino acids in the formation of collagen. In addition, *Aloe vera* is made up of ascorbic acid, zinc, lignins, and saponins, which have a role in increasing collagen synthesis and countervailing collagen breakdown, leading to an increase in the tensile strength of the healing wound [141, 183].

Another mechanism explaining the positive effects of *Aloe vera* on ECM deposition during cutaneous wound repair is that of the MMP-TIMP system. MMPs degrade collagen, while TIMPs inhibit the activity of MMPs.

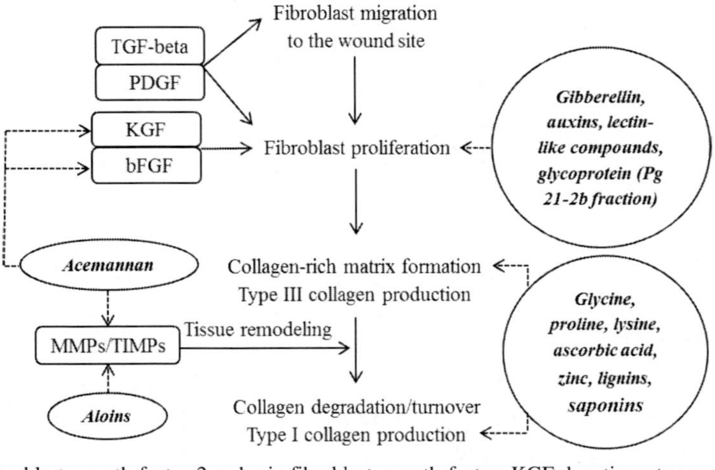

FGF-2, fibroblast growth factor-2 or basic fibroblast growth factor; KGF, keratinocyte growth factor; MMPs, matrix metalloproteinases; PDGF, platelet-derived growth factor; TGF-beta, transforming growth factor-beta; TIMPs, tissue inhibitor metalloproteinases.

Figure 6. Mechanisms underlying *Aloe vera* gel and its components (in bold, italic text) in extracellular matrix formation and remodeling via the stimulation of growth factors.

Barrantes and Guinea have reported that aloe gel and aloins (aloe gel constituents) can inhibit the activity of granulocyte MMPs, likely by destabilizing the enzyme structure [184]. According to Tabandeh et al., MMP-3 and TIMP-2 gene expression is enhanced by the action of mannose-rich Aloe vera polysaccharides [185].

Role of *Aloe Vera* As a Modifier of Factors That Affect Wound Healing

Antimicrobials

The therapeutic effects of *Aloe vera* gel on wound healing can be explained, at least in part, by its antibacterial, antifungal, and antiviral properties in controlling wound infection, which is the most important local factor that retards healing. *In vitro* studies have shown that aloe gel can kill or inhibit the growth of common causative bacteria associated with wound infections, such as *S. aureus, Streptococcus pyogenes, P. aeruginosa, E. coli, Serratia marcescens, Klebsiella pneumonia, Salmonella typhosa,* and *Mycobacterium tuberculosis* [186-192]. The antibacterial activity of aloe has also been demonstrated in the topical treatment of burn wounds in animal experimental studies [193, 194] and in clinical trials [195, 196].

Interestingly, aloe gel, when combined with silver sulfadiazine or mafenide acetate, which are standard topical antibiotic agents used to treat wounds, could accelerate the rate of wound closure in excisional wound rat models, while silver sulfadiazine or mafenide acetate alone delayed this process [197, 198].

However, an experimental study in a thermal burn model in mice did not demonstrate any antibacterial activity of aloe, particularly in third-degree burns in which the wounds were deep and developed severe infections [165]. Another study showed that *Aloe vera* gel applied for 20 min as a first aid treatment for porcine partial-thickness burns, with weekly dressing changes for 6 weeks, did not decrease the microflora in the wound areas [199].

The antimicrobial activities of *Aloe vera* are mediated by at least two mechanisms. First, some ingredients in *Aloe vera* itself might provide direct and indirect antimicrobial activities. Acemannan has been reported to prevent the adherence of *P. aeruginosa* to human lung epithelial cells in culture [200] and to inhibit the replication of Herpes [201] and AIDS viruses [202].

Aloeride, a polysaccharide component from *Aloe vera* gel, has been suggested to possess indirect antimicrobial activity via the stimulation of phagocytic leukocytes [203]. The most potent antibacterial agents against *S. aureus, Streptococcus pyogenes, Bacillus subtilis, and Bacillus cereus* are present in the ethanol and methanol extracts of *Aloe vera gel* and have been identified as p-coumaric acid, ascorbic acid, pyrocatechol, and cinnamic acid [189]. The second mechanism was proposed by Heggers et al. and indicates that *Aloe vera* gel could trigger healing tissues to release some antibacterial factors [204].

Promoter of Oxygenation and Vascularization

Oxygenation and vascularization are enhanced by aloe gel. As previously mentioned in a number of burn wound studies, aloe gel appears to increase blood flow to the injured area by virtue of its ability to restore endothelial function and to stimulate wound angiogenesis, thus improving oxygen access and preventing progressive dermal ischemia [84, 113, 153-157]. The ability of *Aloe vera* to improve oxygenation and vascularization also plays a role in protecting against wound infection, in which tissue hypoxia and ischemia are predisposing factors.

Moisturizer

Another favorable wound healing factor provided by aloe gel is hydration of the wound surface. Aloe gel has a high water content, and it also functions as an occlusive that physically inhibits transepidermal water loss when applied to the skin. Therefore, aloe gel helps to keep wounds moist, enhancing epithelial cell proliferation and migration [205].

Source of Nutrition

In addition to polysaccharides, *Aloe vera* is composed of other active substances that provide benefits for wounds, such as certain amino acids, vitamins (vitamin A, C, and E), and minerals (zinc, copper, iron and magnesium).

Biological/Immunological Modulation of *Aloe Vera* during the Wound Healing Process

In addition to the previously described characteristics, the special and unique therapeutic property of *Aloe vera* that helps to optimize wound healing is its ability to modulate the immune/biological responses. *Aloe vera* has both inhibitory and stimulatory systems, the interactions of which enable cells to adapt and respond properly to injury. Glycoproteins, which are found in the supernatant fraction of the 50% ethanol extract of *Aloe vera* [206], function as the inhibitory system to inhibit the production of free oxygen radicals by polymorphonuclear leukocytes, resulting in anti-inflammatory activity.

Concomitantly, the stimulatory system contains the polysaccharide acemannan, the main component in the precipitate fraction of the 50% ethanol extract of *Aloe vera* [207], which stimulates antibody and cytokine production, as well as immunologically active interleukins, leading to wound healing activity [208].

An example of the biological modulation of aloe is its microcirculatory function during inflammation, as demonstrated by Somboonwong et al. In that particular study, *Aloe vera* gel lyophilized powder could prevent arteriolar vasodilatation and ameliorate the vasoconstriction that occurred during the early and late phases of inflammation after the creation of a second degree burn [84]. This finding indicated that various types of active components in aloe could preserve the internal equilibrium, so-called homeostasis, within the vascular endothelium and surrounding tissues.

Another example is the immunomodulatory effect of aloe on macrophage activation, which plays a considerable role in the wound healing process, including the control of microorganisms and the acceleration of the wound healing rate [208, 209].

Aloe vera and its fractions clearly increased the cell viability of macrophages infected with *Candida albicans in vitro*, according to Farahnejad et al. [210]. The immunomodulatory activity of *Aloe vera* gel was also established *in vivo* by Madan et al., who showed that intraperitoneally injected *Aloe vera* extract could increase the total white blood cell count, humoral immune response and phagocytic activity of peritoneal macrophages [211]. Im et al. also demonstrated that *Aloe vera* gel could function as an immunostimulant because it reduced the growth of *C. albicans* in the spleens and kidneys of normal and diabetic mice when administered orally [212]. The ingredient responsible for this immunomodulatory activity of aloe has been identified as a polysaccharide. It has been shown that acemannan can activate macrophage cytokine production and nitric oxide release [213-215].

These effects have been ascribed in part to the main sugar component of acemannan, called mannose, which binds to the mannose receptors on the surface of macrophages [216]. A subsequent study showed that polysaccharides with molecular weights between 400 and 5 KDa exhibited the most potent macrophage-activating activity *in vitro* [217].

However, aloe has been found to reduce lipopolysaccharide-induced inflammatory cytokine production (IL-8, TNF-alpha, IL-6, and IL-1 beta) in human macrophages and to suppress nitric oxide production by macrophages during inflammation [218, 219].

Based on the above findings, it appears that, in the presence of a combination of the active compounds present in *Aloe vera,* the modulatory systems respond differently, depending on the phases of wound healing, to achieve optimal healing (Figure 7).

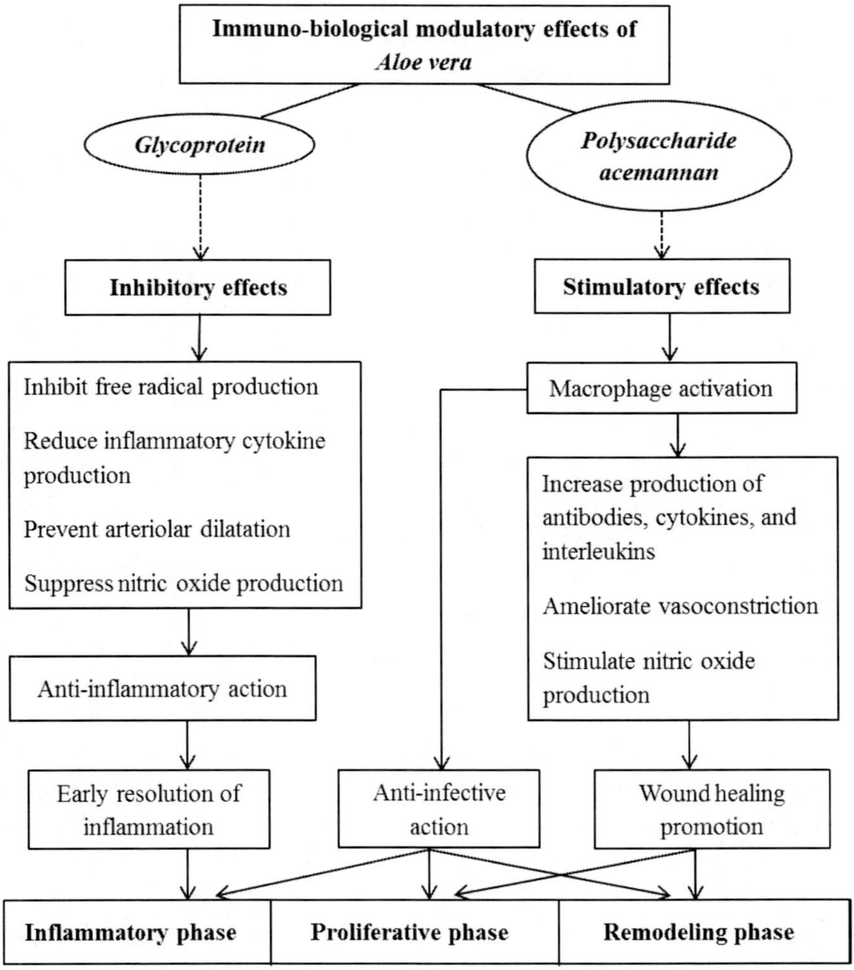

Figure 7. Effects of *Aloe vera* on biological/immunological modulation during different phases of the wound healing process.

Clinical Efficacy of *Aloe Vera* in Wound Healing

A large number of clinical studies have reported the effectiveness of *Aloe vera* in the treatment of cutaneous wounds. This section presents data from systematic reviews of randomized, controlled trials and meta-analyses, which are considered to be the most reliable form of scientific evidence.

The first systematic review on the effectiveness of *Aloe vera* used for any indication was that reported by Vogler and Ernst in 1998 [220]. Among the 10 clinical trials included in this review, two trials undertaken in the US assessed wound healing. One non-randomized, unblinded study compared polyethylene oxide gel with or without *Aloe vera* in 17 patients with acne vulgaris who underwent dermabrasion and received both treatments on each side of their faces. The wounds healed 72 hours faster with *Aloe vera* [109].

Another randomized, unblinded trial was conducted in patients with wound complications after gynecologic surgery and treated with standard wound care with or without *Aloe vera* dermal gel. Those patients who were treated with *Aloe vera* experienced a significantly longer duration to experience complete epithelialization, compared to the standard treatment (83 vs 53 days, respectively) [221].

The clinical efficacy of topical *Aloe vera* in treating burn wounds was reviewed systematically by Maenthaisong et al. in 2007 [222]. This review included four controlled clinical trials (371 patients), two of which were conducted in Thailand [223, 224], while the others were carried out in India [225] and China [226].

All of the studies employed different methodologies in terms of dosage and forms of *Aloe vera* and comparative conventional treatments (aloe fresh mucilage vs sulfadiazine cream, gauze soaked with 85% aloe gel vs petroleum jelly gauze, aloe cream vs framycetin cream, and 1% aloe powder covered with petroleum jelly gauze vs petroleum jelly gauze alone), as well as outcome measurements (time to healing, percentage of the success rate to healing and rate of epithelialization).

The findings showed that *Aloe vera* shortened healing time, with a summary-weighted mean difference of 8.79 days compared to the controls, according to a meta-analysis of the two studies [224, 225].

In addition, aloe tended to increase the success rate of healing and the rate of epithelialization. Topical use of *Aloe vera* was found to be safe because it caused no withdrawal or serious adverse reactions. The authors of this review stated that *Aloe vera* might be effective for first and second degree burns, but well-designed trials with standardization of aloe products are needed to confirm the effectiveness of *Aloe vera* for burn wound healing.

In 2012, the Cochrane Collaboration summarized a systematic review, authored by Dat et al., regarding the effectiveness of *Aloe vera* for the healing of acute and chronic wounds [227]. The primary outcome measurement was either the time to complete wound healing or the proportion of patients with completely healed wounds.

There were seven randomized, controlled clinical trials with a total of 347 patients included from India [225], Iran [228, 229], Thailand [223], and the US [221, 230, 231]. Five trials investigated acute wounds, including burns [223, 225, 228], post-hemorrhoidectomy wounds [229], and excisional skin biopsies [230], while the other two trials pertained to chronic wounds consisting of pressure ulcers [231] and postoperative wounds that healed by secondary intention [221]. In patients with acute wounds, only those undergoing hemorrhoidectomy exhibited a reduction in healing time in response to *Aloe vera* cream containing 0.5% *Aloe vera* gel powder, compared with placebo cream [229]. *Aloe vera* mucilage did not produce a significant difference in burn healing, compared with silver sulfadiazine cream [223]. Similarly, there was no difference in the proportion of participants with completely healed wounds after two weeks of skin biopsy, compared with those who received *Aloe vera* derivative gel dressings containing acemannan and those receiving conventional therapy [230]. In patients with chronic wounds, *Aloe vera* did not appear to display any favorable effects because the acemannan hydrogel dressing did not shorten the pressure ulcer healing time, compared with a saline gauze dressing [231].

In addition, *Aloe vera* dermal gel was combined with a standard management protocol of delayed healing compared with standard management alone in patients with surgical wounds healed by secondary intention [221]. These findings were consistent with previous *Aloe vera* reviews [220, 222]. The authors of this Cochrane review concluded that the existing trial evidence was not sufficient to establish the clinical benefits of *Aloe vera* use for acute and chronic wounds. They recommended the need for properly designed randomized, controlled trials with high methodological quality and validity to assess the effects of *Aloe vera* on wound healing. The outcome measurements should also encompass other related issues, such as the incidence of infection, quality of life, and the financial cost of wound healing.

Later, in 2013, a randomized, controlled trial conducted in Pakistan delineated the efficacy of *Aloe vera* gel compared to 1% sulfadiazine cream in 50 patients with superficial- and partial-thickness burns.

Aloe vera gel was superior to silver sulfadiazine cream in providing rapid wound epithelialization and in reducing pain and treatment costs [232].

Overall, many lines of evidence from preclinical studies have substantiated the therapeutic effects of *Aloe vera,* as well as its underlying mechanisms in wound healing. However, the clinical efficacy of aloe remains to be established.

Centella Asiatica and Its Mechanisms in Wound Healing

Centella asiatica belongs to the Araliaceae family based on genetic evidence, and it was also previously categorized in the Apiaceae (Umbelliferae) family. The scientific name is *Centella asiatica* (Linn.) Urban, and its synonyms include *Centella coriacea* Nannfd., *Hydrocotyle asiatica* L., *Hydrocotyle lunata* Lam., and *Trisanthus cochinchinesis* Lour. It is commonly known as gotu kola, and Asiatic or Indian pennywort. *C. asiatica* is a slender herb that is native to tropical and sub-tropical regions, and it grows particularly abundantly in moist areas of Southeast Asia, Africa, Australia, Central America, and Madagascar. It has long, prostrate stems with thin, spade-shaped leaves and short clusters of sessile, white flowers [233].

According to plant chemical assays, *C. asiatica* is composed of various compounds, such as triterpenes, essential oils (caryophyllene, farnesol, and elemene), flavonoids (quercetin and kaempferol, catechin, rutin, and naringin), polysaccharides, polyyne-alkene, amino acids, fatty acids, sesquiterpenes, alkaloids, sterols, carotenoids, tannin, chlorophyll, pectin, and inorganic salts. The major chemical constituents of *C. asiatica* are triterpenes, including triterpenic acids and their respective phenolic glycosides, such as asiatic acid, asiaticoside, madecassic acid, madecassoside, brahmic acid, brahmoside, brahminoside, thankuniside, isothankuniside, centelloside, madasiatic acid, centic acid, cenellic acid, betulinic acid, and indocentic acid, among others. [234]. Of these constituents, asiatic acid, asiaticoside, madecassic acid, and madecassoside are considered to be the most important bioactive compounds.

C. asiatica has been long known for its therapeutic use in wounds, burns, various skin conditions and neurological and gastrointestinal disorders, in Ayurvedic medicine, traditional Chinese medicine, and traditional Southeast Asian medicine. The plant is included in the drug lists within the pharmacopoeias of many countries, such as Germany, India, and the People's

Republic of China [233]. In India and Pakistan, crushed leaves are topically applied to treat wounds or skin ulcers [233]. In Thailand, *C. asiatica* is included in the Thai Fundamental Public Health Drug List as a wound healing agent in the formulation of extract cream [106].

Many scientific data have supported the efficacy of *C. asiatica* in the treatment of wounds and burns, as well as in hypertrophic scar prevention. A clinical study was conducted in 22 patients with chronic skin ulcers using a 1% cream of the extracted triterpenoids without a placebo control.

It was found that the average healing rates were 24%, 37%, and 47% after one, two, and three weeks of treatment, respectively [235]. In another prospective, randomized, controlled study enrolling 200 diabetic wound patients, the oral administration of *C. asiatica* capsules (300 mg of extracted asiaticoside per day) appeared to promote wound healing and to suppress scar formation without any serious side effects during the course of a 21-day therapy, compared to placebo [236]. However, there have been no systematic reviews documenting the clinical efficacy of *C. asiatica* in the treatment of wounds.

In experimental animal studies, *C. asiatica* extract and its triterpenoid compounds have been reported to be effective when applied topically in various wound models, such as acute radiation dermatitis, punch, incision, excision, dead space wound and burn wound models [80, 237-239], or when administered orally in a burn wound model [240].

The efficacy of *C. asiatica* in wound healing can vary with the types of plant extracts used and thus with the major constituents yielded, producing different effects during various phases of wound healing. Somboonwong et al. examined the effects of the topical application of four different extracts of *C. asiatica*, namely hexane, ethyl acetate, methanol, and aqueous extracts, on the healing of partial-thickness burn wounds in rats. Thin layer chromatography profiling of the four extracts was also performed to identify the major active compounds. All of the extracts were found to increase the extent of healing, but at different monitored time points. The ethyl acetate extract, which contained asiatic acid, resulted in the earliest onset of healing on day 3, and the healing effect was sustained throughout the 14-day experimental period. Significant effects were later observed with the use of hexane extract consisting of beta-sitosterol on days 10 and 14, while methanol extract, consisting of asiaticoside and madecassoside, and aqueous extract, which lacks the identifiable substances mentioned above but which is known to have a high flavonoid content, provided effects on day 14. However, all of the extracts resulted in a comparable extent of wound healing on day 14 [80]. These observations indicate that each active substance present in *C. asiatica* could play a different role during various phases of wound healing.

Role of *C. Asiatica* in the Suppression of Wound Inflammation

The effects of *C. asiatica* on the inhibition of wound inflammation have been reported after burn injury. Using a partial-thickness burn wound rat model, the aforementioned study of Somboonwong et al. showed that, after three days of wound infliction, the untreated wounds were swollen and bruised, while those locally treated with *C. asiatica* extracts (hexane, ethyl acetate, methanol, and aqueous extracts) exhibited mild swelling and dry wound surfaces. Furthermore, upon histological examination on day 14 post-wounding, the untreated wounds still had some inflammation; however, in the treated wounds, no inflammation was observed. Among the extracts studied, the ethyl acetate extract of *C. asiatica*, which mainly contained asiatic acid, appeared to elicit an early anti-inflammatory effect, in addition to causing a rapid onset of healing, as described previously [80].

Another study, conducted by Liu et al., also revealed a beneficial effect of madecassoside, the major triterpene isolated from *C. asiatica*, on burn wound healing when administered orally in mice, and decreases in inflammatory cell infiltration and nitric oxide were observed in the burned skin tissues [240].

Information on microcirculatory changes to demonstrate the anti-inflammatory effects of *C. asiatica* during the wound healing process remains lacking. However, in other conditions, such as chronic venous insufficiency and microangiopathy, the results obtained from a systematic review conducted by Chong and Aziz seemed to suggest that *C. asiatica* improved tissue microcirculation in terms of the transcutaneous partial pressure of oxygen and carbon dioxide, capillary permeability, and venoarteriolar response.

However, the clinical relevance of these results remains inconclusive due to the inadequate reporting of the included studies and their unclear risk of bias [241].

The suppressive effects of *C. asiatica* and its components on wound inflammation are mainly due to the inhibition of prostaglandins, kinins, histamine, pro-inflammatory cytokines, and pro-inflammatory enzymes, as well as antioxidant activity and the stabilization of lysosomal enzymes (Figure 8).

Antiprostaglandin Activities

C. asiatica has been shown to possess anti-inflammatory properties by inhibiting COX and subsequent prostaglandin production. Somchit et al. revealed that an intraperitoneal injection of the aqueous extract of *C. asiatica* (2, 4, and 10 mg/kg) elicited a dose-dependent anti-inflammatory effect on PGE2-induced paw edema in rats, similar to the NSAID mefenamic acid. In the same study, *C. asiatica* (10, 30, 100, and 300 mg/kg) also exerted antinociceptive activity in mice, similarly to aspirin but less potent than morphine [242].

The constituents of *C. asiatica* that exhibit antiprostaglandin activity have been documented to be the triterpenes and their glycosides. In accord with Yun et al. and Won et al., asiatic acid and madecassic acid inhibited lipopolysaccharide-induced PGE2 production and COX-2 expression in RAW 264.7 macrophage cells through NF-κB inactivation [243, 244].

In a study reported by Nurlaily et al., asiaticoside and madecassoside also suppressed both COX-1 and COX-2 activities, along with PGE2 production *in vitro*. In addition, when the different extracts of *C. asiatica* were compared, the ethanol and methanol extracts contained larger amounts of these two triterpene glycosides, and they exerted stronger anti-inflammatory activity than the aqueous extract [245]. However, asiatic acid and madecassic acid have been found to possess more potent antiprostaglandin activity than asiaticoside or madecassoside [243, 244].

Antikinin/Antihistamine Activity

There is indirect evidence indicating that *C. asiatica* might inhibit the activity of histamine or kinins. George et al. found that ethanolic and aqueous extracts of *C. asiatica* prevented the degranulation of mast cells, which release histamine during inflammation. The results of that study also revealed that the ethanolic extract of *C. asiatica* (100 mg/kg) administered orally could reduce paw edema provoked by carrageenan in rats [246].

In another study reported by Saha et al. in rats, an inhibitory effect on carrageenan-induced paw inflammation was demonstrated for methanol extract (200 mg/kg) but not for chloroform extract, with maximum inhibition observed at 2 h. Considering that carrageenan-induced inflammation shows biphasic responses through the release of histamine, serotonin, and kinins during the first phase and prostaglandins during the second phase, Saha et al. proposed that the anti-inflammatory activity of *C. asiatica* is likely mediated by inhibition of the liberation of histamine or kinins [247].

Inhibition of Pro-Inflammatory Cytokine/Enzyme Activity

In the studies reported Yun et al. and Won et al. mentioned above, PGE2 inhibition, asiatic acid and madecassic acid exert their anti-inflammatory effects by inhibiting the expression of the pro-inflammatory cytokines IL-6, IL-1β, and TNF-α, as well as the pro-inflammatory enzyme iNOS, via NF-κB inactivation in RAW 264.7 macrophages [243, 244].

Asiatic acid is regarded as the most powerful constituent of *C. asiatica* in stimulating the expression of TNFAIP6, a hyaladherin that is involved in ECM remodeling and that possesses anti-inflammatory properties, as stated in a study by Coldren et al. [248]. These effects of asiatic acid account for the early wound healing ability and anti-inflammatory activity of the ethyl acetate extract of *C. asiatica,* as noted previously in the study by Somboonwong et al. [80].

Antioxidant Activity

C. asiatica possesses antioxidant activity, which is known to reduce inflammation. The antioxidant potential of *C. asiatica* is due to the presence of asiaticoside, madecassoside, flavonoids, polyphenol, carotene, tannin, and vitamin C [245, 249, 250].

Stabilization of the Lysosomal Membrane

An *in vitro* study performed by Chippada et al. affirmed that the human red blood cell membrane, which is analogous to that of the lysosome, was stabilized by the methanolic extract of *C. asiatica* [251]. Therefore, it is possible that *C. asiatica* aids in limiting the inflammatory response, at least in part, by stabilizing the lysosomal membrane. These effects result in inhibition of the release of lysosomal enzymes by activated neutrophils, thus preventing further tissue inflammation and damage.

Role of *C. Asiatica* in Wound Angiogenesis

Terpene glycosides and beta-sitosterol are the principal compounds responsible for stimulating wound angiogenesis (Figure 9). Shukla et al. showed that asiaticoside isolated from *C. asiatica* could enhance wound healing by stimulating angiogenesis. Asiaticoside produces new capillary formation in the CAM model, with the greatest response observed using a disk concentration of 40 mcg [252]. The molecular pathways underlying this angiogenic effect were examined by Coldren et al., using a fibroblast cell culture model system. The results revealed that the titrated extract of *C. asiatica* (TECA), which consisted of asiatic acid (30%), madecassic acid (30%), and asiaticoside (40%), affected the expression of genes involved in angiogenesis by inducing genes encoding pro-angiogenic factors, such as plasminogen activator inhibitor-2 (PAI2), VEGF, FGF1, and FGF2, while reducing the expression of anti-angiogenic thrombospondin [248]. This phenomenon shifted the balance toward an increase in angiogenesis.

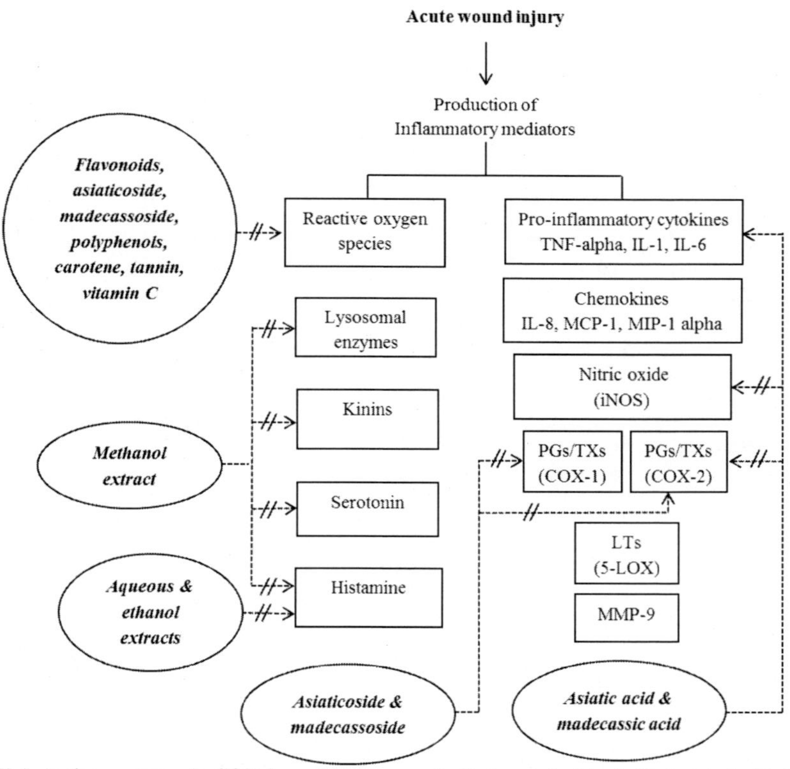

COX-1, cyclooxygenase-1; COX-2, cyclooxygenase-2; IL-1, interleukin-1; IL-6, interleukin-6; IL-8, interleukin-8; iNOS, inducible nitric oxide synthase; 5-LOX, 5-lipoxygenase; LTs, leukotrienes; MCP-1, monocyte chemoattractant protein-1; MIP-1 alpha, macrophage-inflammatory protein-1 alpha; MMP-9, matrix metalloproteinase-9; PGs, prostaglandins; TNF-alpha, tumor necrosis factor-alpha; TXs, thromboxanes.

Figure 8. Inhibition by *Centella asiatica* and its components (in italic, bold text) of the inflammatory mediators produced during wound inflammation. Asiaticoside and madecassoside reduce the expression of the pro-inflammatory cytokines iNOS, and COX-2 by inhibiting nuclear factor-kappa-B activation. Enzymes that stimulate the synthesis of nitric oxide, PGs/TXs, and LTs are shown in parentheses.

Additionally, Kimura et al. reported a facilitating action of topical asiaticoside at low doses of 10^{-8} to 10^{-12}% (w/w) in burn wound healing, by promoting angiogenesis through an increase in the expression of MCP-1 and IL-1-beta, which enhance VEGF production [253].

In addition to asiaticoside, madecassoside also facilitated angiogenesis in burn wound healing in mice and stimulated endothelial cell growth in a rat aortic ring assay, as demonstrated by the previously mentioned study reported by Liu et al. [240]. However, the mechanism of action underlying the angiogenic effect of madecassoside remains poorly understood.

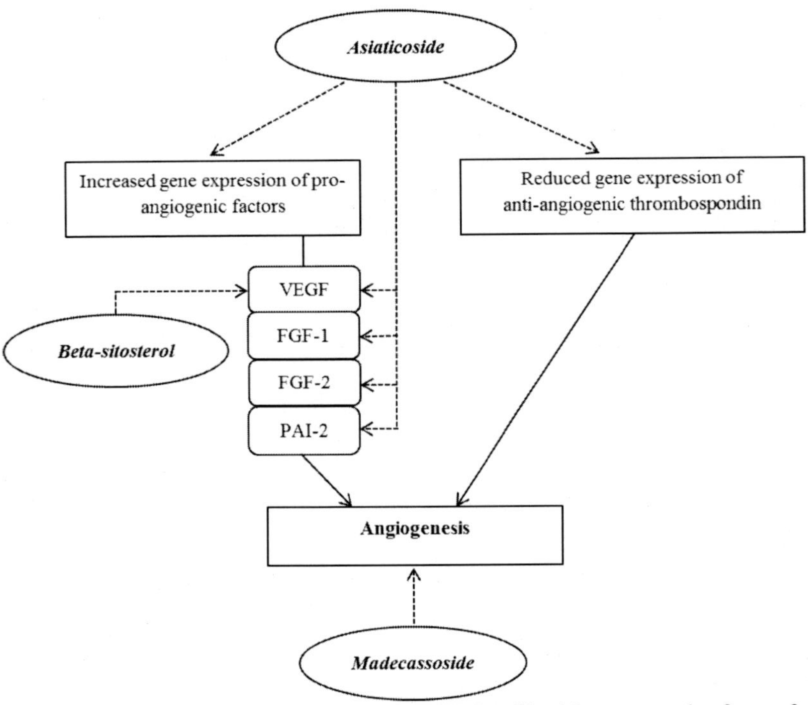

FGF-1, fibroblast growth factor-1; FGF-2, fibroblast growth factor-2; PAI-2, plasminogen-activating factor-2; VEGF, vascular endothelial growth factor.

Figure 9. Effects of asiaticoside, beta-sitosterol, and madecassoside on the stimulation of wound angiogenesis.

Beta-sitosterol is another compound that is known to possess potent angiogenic activity, as previously described in the *Aloe vera* section [161, 162]. It being a major constituent of the hexane extract of *C. asiatica* partially explains the observation of Somboonwong et al. that significant healing of burn wounds in rats treated with the hexane extract of *C. asiatica* occurred later on day 10 and 14 post-wounding, corresponding to the proliferative phase of wound healing, during which angiogenesis occurs [80].

Role of *C. Asiatica* in Fibroblast Proliferation, Matrix Formation and Remodeling

C. asiatica has been well documented to play a positive role in ECM formation and remodeling during wound repair. A large number of *in vivo* experiments have demonstrated an increase in the synthesis of collagen, hydroxyproline or glycosaminoglycan or enhancement of the tensile strength of wounds following the administration of *C. asiatica* extracts [80, 239, 254, 255], as well as triterpenoid compounds, including asiatic acid [238], madecassic acid [238], siaticoside [238, 252], and madecassoside [240], In addition to the effect on normal wound healing, similar results were obtained in delayed healing models, such as dexamethasone-suppressed wound healing [239] and diabetic wound healing [252].

Furthermore, *in vitro* studies using cultured human skin fibroblasts have substantiated an increase in fibronectin, the principal noncollagenous matrix glycoprotein in stromal connective tissue, in addition to collagen [256, 257].

In the study by Hashim, exceptional increases in collagen and fibronectin were observed when *C. asiatica* was combined with glycolic acid and vitamins A, C, and E [257]. Regarding impact on wound remodeling, Suguna et al. demonstrated that an alcoholic extract of *C. asiatica,* administered orally or topically, resulted in high stability of acid-soluble collagen and increases in aldehyde content and tensile strength in healing rat wounds, indicating swifter and improved maturation and crosslinking of collagen.

Research has attempted to elucidate the active compounds in *C. asiatica* that are responsible for collagen production and wound remodeling. A comparison of the three triterpenes (asiatic acid, madecassic acid, and asiaticoside) revealed that asiatic acid and asiaticoside were the most active triterpenes in stimulating ECM accumulation, with asiaticoside producing a favorable stimulation of collagen synthesis [238]. In one study, asiaticoside (30 μM) stimulated the mRNA and protein production of type I and type III collagen in human dermal fibroblasts *in vitro* [258]. Another *in vitro* study reported that only madecassoside possessed the ability to induce type III collagen production. In addition, both asiaticoside and madecassoside could stimulate the synthesis of type I collagen, which replaces the type III collagen produced during the early phase of wound healing to replenish the normal collagen composition during the remodeling phase [259]. A comparative study of the four main compounds by Wu et al. showed that asiaticoside and madecassoside, rather than asiatic acid and madecassic acid, could enhance type I and type III collagen synthesis and that madecassoside exhibited a more potent effect than asiaticoside in promoting type III collagen synthesis [260].

C. asiatica increases the accumulation of ECM in dermal tissues through multiple mechanisms (Figure 10). The first mechanism is skin the fibroblast activation attributed to asiaticoside, which proceeds simply by enhancing the fibroblast activity related to wound healing.

Using a wound closure seeding model, Lee et al. revealed that asiaticoside increased the migration rates, initial adhesion, and proliferation of normal human skin fibroblasts. In addition, it has been proposed that asiaticoside might provide a therapeutic benefit when it is incorporated into an artificial dermis because its potential in activating initial skin cell adhesion is expected to cause rapid and secure attachment of the transplanted epidermis [261].

The mechanism responsible for the promotion of human fibroblast proliferation by asiaticoside is partly due to up-regulation of the expression of genes encoding cell proliferation and cell-cycle progression [258]. In contrast, Wu et al. showed no evidence of the stimulating effects of asiaticoside, madecassoside, asiatic acid, or madecassic acid at concentrations of 1, 3, and 10 μM on the proliferation of skin fibroblasts [260].

Second, triterpene extracts from *C. asiatica* trigger the expression of hyaladherin (proteins that bind to hyaluronan, which is a non-collagenous component of the extracellular matrix) and cytokines, including PAI-2 and TGF-beta, as reported by Coldren et al. [248].

Increased PAI-2 results in a decrease in collagen degradation [262, 263], and increased TGF-beta directly stimulates fibroblasts to synthesize collagen and fibronectin and also partially induces them to differentiate into myofibroblasts, to facilitate wound contraction [264]. However, in one study, the expression levels of collagen and fibronectin genes were not directly affected [264].

Among the three TGF-beta isotypes secreted from macrophages, TGF-beta-1 is mostly related to wound healing. Binding of TGF-beta-1 to TGF-beta type I and type II receptors leads to the phosphorylation of receptor-regulated SMADs (R-Smads), namely Smad 2 and Smad 3. This phenomenon is followed by heterodimer formation with common Smad (co-Smad), Smad 4 and Smad 7 and translocation to the nucleus to mediate downstream gene expression, resulting in profibrogenesis. Smad 7 is an inhibitory Smad (I-Smad) in TGF-beta/Smad signaling transduction.

Asiaticoside and madecassoside have been shown to induce type I collagen production in normal human skin fibroblasts via the activation of the TGF-beta/Smad pathway [260, 265].

Lee et al. demonstrated that this activation occurred independently of TGF-beta receptor I and that the activation, in turn, induced the phosphorylation of Smad 2 and Smad 3, together with the binding of Smad 3 and Smad 4 [265]. Moreover, Wu et al. discovered that asiaticoside and madecassoside increased type I and type III collagen synthesis by skin fibroblasts via the TGF-beta/Smad pathway, whereas neither asiatic acid nor madecassic acid affected this process [260]. Moreover, the two glycosides were found to increase the mRNA expression of TGF-beta receptor II and the phosphorylation of Smad 3 and to elevate TGF-beta-1 levels in skin tissues, thus improving the speed and quality of full-thickness burn wound healing [260].

Another mechanism underlying the facilitating effects of *C. asiatica* on wound repair is mediated via the antioxidant activity of some compounds, such as asiaticoside, madecassoside, and flavonoids [80, 240, 249, 266]. During inflammation, reactive oxygen species generated by phagocytic leukocytes not only amplify the inflammatory response but also promote cytotoxicity. In addition to enhanced free radical formation, there is impairment of antioxidant mechanisms because the activities of antioxidant enzymes, such as superoxide dismutase, are reduced after a burn injury. Antioxidants help to control wound oxidative stress and thus prevent DNA damage, augmenting wound healing. Asiaticoside and madecassoside have been reported to reduce wound oxidative stress by modulating antioxidant levels and free radical production. Shukla et al. demonstrated that the topical application of 0.2% asiaticoside elevated the levels of enzymatic and non-enzymatic antioxidants, including superoxide dismutase, catalase, glutathione peroxidase, vitamin E, and ascorbic acid, while reducing lipid peroxide levels in wound tissues at 7 days but not at 14 days post-wounding [266]. Liu et al. demonstrated that oral administration of madecassoside (12 and 24 mg/kg) decreased malondialdehyde content while increasing the reduced glutathione and hydroxyproline in burn wound tissues [240]. Moreover, Somboonwong et al. suggested that a high content of flavonoids as antioxidants, present in the aqueous extract of *C. asiatica,* might be responsible for the wound healing activity observed during the late stage of this process (after 14 days) [80]. This finding was supported by Nurlaily et al., who reported that, among three different extracts of *C. asiatica* (methanol, ethanol, and aqueous extracts), the aqueous extract displayed the greatest antioxidant potential [245].

Whether MMPs and TIMPs, which contribute to collagen degradation and consequent ECM deposition during the granulation tissue formation stage and the remodeling period, are influenced by *C. asiatica* remains controversial.

Wu et al. demonstrated no alteration in the ratio of MMP-1 to TIMP-1 in cultured human skin fibroblasts in the presence of asiaticoside, madecassoside, asiatic acid or madecassic acid [260].

However, Nema et al. noted that asiaticoside exhibited an inhibitory effect on MMP-1, as well as on hyaluronidase and elastase *in vitro* [267].

Role of *C. Asiatica* in Wound Re-Epithelialization

Using *C. asiatica* and its constituents, better re-epithelialization of wounds has been observed in several experimental studies.

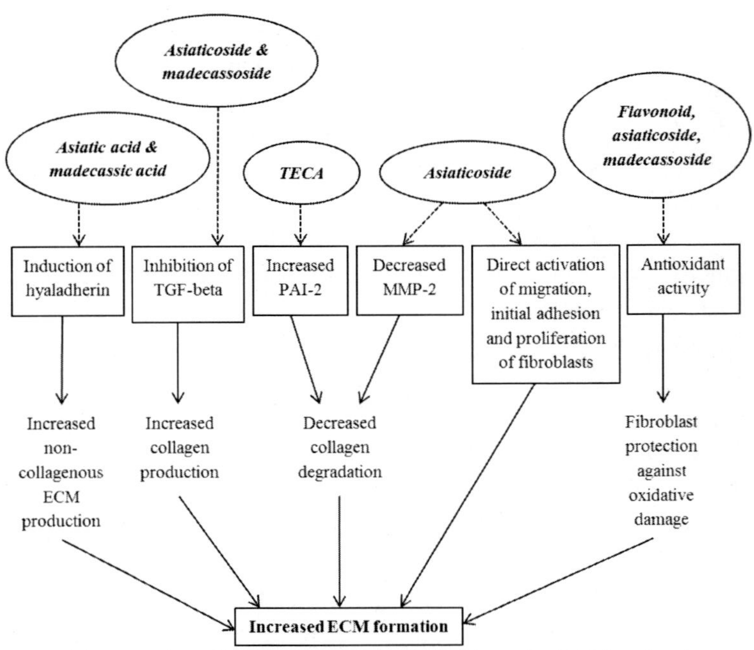

ECM, extracellular matrix; MMP-2, matrix metalloproteinase-2; PAI-2, plasminogen-activator inhibitor-2; TECA, titrated extract of *C. asiatica* (a mixture of 40% asiaticoside, 30% asiatic acid, and 30% madecassic acid); TGF-beta, transforming growth factor-beta.

Figure 10. Mechanisms of action of *Centella asiatica* and its components in the increased extracellular matrix formation that occurs during wound healing.

The following examples were provided: 1) topical formulations (ointment, cream, and gel) of the aqueous extract of *C. asiatica* on open wounds in rats by Sunikumar et al. [255]; 2) topical and oral administration of an alcoholic extract of *C. asiatica* on rat dermal wounds by Suguna et al. (1996) [254]; 3) topical application of an ethanolic extract on rats using incision, excision, and dead space wound models by Shetty et al. [239]; 4) topical application of *C. asiatica* extracts (hexane, ethyl acetate, methanol, and aqueous extracts) on rat burn wounds by Somboonwong et al. (2012) [80]; 5) topical application of 0.2% and 0.4% asiaticoside solutions over punch wounds in guinea pigs and diabetic rats, respectively, by Shukla et al. [252]; and 6) oral madecassoside (6, 12, and 24 mg/kg) in mice subjected to burn injuries by Liu et al. [240].

Asiaticoside has been shown to influence the epithelialization process via at least two mechanisms. First, it stimulated the cells of the Malphigian layer, the deepest part of the epidermis in which mitotic activity occurs, and it activated keratinization, as demonstrated histologically in the porcine epidermis by the study reported by May [268]. Second, it increased the migration and the initial adhesion of keratinocytes in the epidermal layers of the skin in an *in vitro* wound healing model, according to Lee et al. [261]. However, it did not affect keratinocyte proliferation in cell proliferation assays [261].

Madecassoside enhances the re-epithelialization of burn wounds in mice, as previously mentioned; however, little is known about the underlying mechanism. Overall, it has been noted that additional studies are needed to elucidate the biomolecular mechanisms responsible for the effect of *C. asiatica* on wound re-epithelialization.

Role of *C. Asiatica* in Improvement of Abnormal Scars

Hypertrophic and keloid scars are abnormal scars that result from a pathological response to skin injury, leading to poor functional and cosmetic outcomes. They are characterized by excessive fibrosis (excessive collagen synthesis and deposition) with disorganized collagen, an altered ratio of type I to type III collagen, and a delay or blockade of wound maturation process [3]. Hypertrophic scarring is also related to prolongation of the inflammatory process, and the inhibition of inflammation can reduce scar formation. The molecular pathogenesis of keloid formation implicates mainly TGF-beta, with increases in the expression of TGF-beta-1 and TGF-beta-2 and a decrease in the expression of TGF-beta-3 [269].

Overexpression of TGF-beta 1, in addition to increasing collagen synthesis and fibroblast proliferation, could decrease the degradation of collagen by suppressing MMP-1 and PA and by activating TIMP-1 and PAI. It is interesting to note that scarless healing, as observed in the fetus during early gestation, is caused by different responses to wounding compared to scar healing: a reduced inflammatory response, lower TGF-beta 1 and TGF-beta 2, and higher TGF-beta 3 [270].

The most interesting beneficial effects of *C. asiatica* might be the phenomena of hypertrophic scarring prevention and reduction. Widgerow et al. suggested that scar control could be achieved by three modalities: wound support to reduce the tension on a scar; hydration; and hastened maturity [271]. Based on these modalities, they formulated a scar management program using microporous tape to support the scar, in combination with Alpha Centella® cream consisting of two components: *Bulbine frutescens* extract to provide hydration and to prevent bacterial infection; and *C. asiatica* extract, containing asiatic acid, madecassic acid, and asiaticoside, to accelerate healing. This product was employed in 106 patients during the first 6 to 8 weeks of the postoperative period. Observations after a minimum of 6 months of follow-up revealed accelerated scar maturity and satisfactory scar appearance, with excellent patient compliance and no adverse drug reactions related to the cream preparation. The preventive effect of *C. asiatica* on scar formation has been proposed to result from its ability to promote scar maturity and to inhibit wound inflammation.

For readily established hypertrophic and keloid scars, recent research has focused on identifying the responsible constituents and on clarifying the underlying molecular mechanisms, particularly those involving inhibition of the TGF-beta/Smad pathway [272-275].

Asiaticoside has been reported to be effective for the management of hypertrophic scars and keloids [272-274, 276]. Asiaticoside prevented new scar formation by reducing fibrosis in wounds [277]. Zhang et al. showed that the topical application of asiaticoside on post-burn hypertrophic scars resulted in down-regulation of TGF-beta 1 mRNA and TIMP 1 expression and up-regulation of TGF-beta-3 expression, but it did not affect MMP expression. Moreover, it had the ability to break down type I collagen products in post-burn hypertrophic scars, as evidenced by a decrease in type I collagen expression [272]. Xie et al. explored the antiscarring effect of asiaticoside and its mechanism using a rabbit ear model with a hypertrophic scar. Treatment with 0.5% and 1% asiaticoside solutions produced a remarkable reduction in scarring.

The underlying mechanism is mediated by a decrease in the expression of TGF-beta-1 and an increase in the expression of the inhibitory Smad7, with no observed effects on Smad2 [273]. Tang et al. showed that asiaticoside decreased the proliferation of keloid-derived fibroblasts, in contrast to its effect on normal skin healing. They also confirmed that asiaticoside inhibited type I and type II collagen expression and TGF-beta/Smad signaling via the induction of Smad7 and suppression of TGF-beta receptor-1 and TGF-beta receptor-2 in keloid fibroblasts [274].

Asiatic acid impedes keloid formation by inhibiting TGF-beta/Smad signaling. Based on the observations of Bian et al., asiatic acid does not interfere with cell proliferation, but it can inhibit cell invasion and collagen synthesis in keloid fibroblasts stimulated with TGF-beta-1. Moreover, asiatic acid can inhibit collagen type I and PAI-1 expression, indicating that it affects the reduction of collagen production and increases collagen degradation. In addition, it suppresses Smad 2/3 phosphorylation while elevating Smad 7 protein levels in TGF-beta 1-treated keloid fibroblasts. The underlying mechanism proceeds via PPAR-gamma activation [275].

The unique characteristic of keloid scars is their expansion beyond the site of the original injury due to the remarkable migratory activity of fibroblasts. Song et al. noted that madecassoside could diminish keloid formation by suppressing the migration of keloid-derived fibroblasts, which originate from human earlobe keloids, and this process was mediated by the p38 kinase and PI3K signaling pathways [278].

Role of *C. Asiatica* As a Modifier of Factors That Affect Wound Healing

Antimicrobials

Several extracts of *C. asiatica* have been reported to possess antibacterial, antifungal, and antiviral activities *in vitro*. Hexane and ethyl acetate extracts of *C. asiatica* inhibited the growth of Gram-positive *Bacillus subtilis* and Gram-negative *P. aeruginosa, P. cichorii,* and *E. coli* in the disc diffusion test [279]. Petroleum ether, ethanol, and chloroform extracts were very active against Gram-positive *B. subtilis* and *S. aureus* and Gram-negative *Proteus vulgaris* and *E. coli* [280]. The methanol extract was shown to be moderately effective against *S. aureus and* methicillin-resistant *S. aureus* [281]. Asiaticoside, when coupled with liposomes, was more effective than free asiaticoside against *M. tuberculosis* and *M. leprae* [282].

Petroleum ether, ethanol, chloroform, n-hexane, and aqueous extracts displayed antifungal activity against *A. niger* and *C. albicans* [280]. The aqueous extract of *C. asiatica* was also found to possess antiviral activity against type 2 Herpes simplex virus [279].

Little information is available regarding the therapeutic efficacy of *C. asiatica* against wound infection or the responsible active ingredients and their mechanisms of action. However, based on the above *in vitro* studies, the active ingredients of *C. asiatica* that exert antimicrobial effects against bacteria commonly detected in infected wounds, such as *S. aureus, P. vulgaris, P. aeruginosa,* and *E. coli,* appear to reside in the hexane, ethyl acetate, petroleum ether, ethanol, methanol, and chloroform extracts. These findings provide a basis for further investigations of the role of *C. asiatica* as an anti-infective agent for wound infections.

Curcuma Longa and Its Mechanisms in Wound Healing

Curcuma longa is a rhizomatous perennial herb of the Zingiberaceae (ginger) family. The scientific name is *Curcuma longa* (Linn.), and its synonyms are *Curcuma domestica* Valeton., *C. rotunda* L., *C. xanthorrhiza* Naves, and *Amomum curcuma* Jacq. The common name for *C. longa* is turmeric. The plant is geographically distributed throughout the tropics and is particularly cultivated in India, China, Indonesia, Thailand and tropical regions of Africa. It has fleshy, oblong, palmate rhizomes (roots) that are orange-yellow to orange internally, with large lanceolate leaves and white-to-light-green bracts subtending pale yellow flowers [233].

C. longa has been widely used as a spice and coloring agent in Southern and Southeastern Asian cuisine, as well as in cosmetics and drugs. Similar to *Aloe vera and C. asiatica*, *C. longa* has a long history of use in Ayurvedic and Chinese medicine. As described in pharmacopoeias and in traditional systems of medicine, it is used to treat a wide variety of diseases, including peptic ulcers, inflammatory conditions, skin diseases, pain, and wounds. For example, it is used as a home remedy to relieve pain and inflammation by the local application of a paste formulation of the powdered rhizome of *C. longa* mixed with slaked lime or by application in poultices [233].

The principal chemical constituents of the rhizome *C. longa* include the three yellow-colored curcuminoids, namely curcumin (or diferuloylmethane)

(70-76%), demethoxycurcumin (16%), and bisdemethoxycurcumin (8%). In addition, it is composed of pale yellow to orange-yellow volatile oils (turmerone, curcumene, atlantone, and zingiberene), sugars, proteins, and resins. Among the three curcuminoids, curcumin is the best studied and is referred to as the most active component of *C. longa*. Curcumin has been claimed to possess anti-inflammatory, antioxidant, anticancer, antimicrobial, and wound healing activities [233].

Research has demonstrated that curcumin is an effective wound healing agent for both normal, as well as delayed healing, wounds in different animal models. Using a punch wound model in rats and guinea pigs, Sidhu et al. reported that curcumin accelerated the rate of wound closure and that the treated wounds displayed re-epithelialization, the migration of various cells including macrophages, fibroblasts, and myofibroblasts, angiogenesis, and collagen deposition to greater extents than untreated wounds [283]. In a rat burn wound model, according to Kulac et al., topical treatment with curcumin also accelerated healing and improved inflammatory cell numbers, collagen deposition, hydroxyproline levels, angiogenesis, granulation tissue formation and epithelialization [284]. Interestingly, Singer et al. showed that the treatment of full-thickness burns with curcumin, either administered orally prior to injury and three days after injury or given intravenously 1 and 24 hours after injury, could curtail the progression of the ischemic zone to complete necrosis [285, 286].

Curcumin has been found to help promote the impaired wound healing caused by diabetic conditions or irradiation. Sidhu et al. noticed that the oral and topical application of curcumin could enhance the re-epithelialization, neovascularization, cell migration, and collagen content of full-thickness cutaneous punch wounds inflicted in diabetic animals [287]. In a series of studies conducted by Jagetia and Rajanikant, the effects of curcumin on excisional wounds in mice exposed to gamma radiation were investigated. Pretreatment with curcumin ameliorated the deteriorating healing of irradiated wounds, manifesting prolonged wound contraction and healing times, reductions in collagen, hexosamine, DNA, and nitric oxide synthesis, and diminished fibroblast and vascular densities [288-291]. In incisional skin wounds generated with a carbon dioxide laser, another example of delayed healing wounds, López-Jornet et al. demonstrated that topical curcumin induced early wound re-epithelialization after seven days, although no significant effects on inflammatory processes were detected [292].

Due to the low bioavailability and low *in vivo* stability of curcumin, increasing numbers of studies have attempted to develop improved transdermal delivery vehicles to improve its efficacy in wound healing. Curcumin-incorporated collagen matrix films could improve the quality of wound healing and could also provide additional antioxidant activity, compared to normal collagen films [293]. The encapsulation of curcumin with poly(lactic-co-glycolic acid) (PLGA) polymer nanoparticles offers advantages for light protection, water solubility and the sustained release of curcumin. These PLGA-curcumin nanoparticles have exhibited two-fold greater wound healing activity than curcumin or PLGA alone, with better re-epithelialization, granulation tissue formation and anti-inflammatory effects in a full-thickness excisional wound mouse model [294]. A biodegradable hydrogel system, containing curcumin-loaded polymeric micelles, provided good tissue adhesiveness and sustained curcumin release. Its application as a wound dressing enhanced the tensile strength of incision wounds and improved the collagen content, granulation tissue formation, and wound maturity of full-thickness excision wounds [295]. A curcumin-loaded oleic acid-based polymeric bandage elicited superior wound healing potency and reduced the inflammatory response, compared to a void bandage or cotton gauze in a rat model [296]. Various wound dressing formulations, utilizing a chitosan-alginate biodegradable sponge loaded with curcumin [297], a curcumin-beta-cyclodextrin-loaded sponge [298], nano-curcumin combined with chitosan-alginate hydrogel [299], and curcumin-loaded poly(epsilon-caprolactone)-poly(ethylene glycol)-poly(epsilon-caprolactone) (PCEC) fibrous mats [300], have also provided promising results for wound healing.

In addition, Castangia et al. showed that curcumin bionanovesicles could greatly diminish chemical-induced inflammation as measured by myeloperoxidase activity, and they produced considerable epithelialization of full-thickness skin lesions in mice [301].

The above evidence indicates that curcumin plays a role in every phase of the tissue repair and wound healing processes that involve inflammation, granulation, and remodeling of the tissue. The possible mechanisms underlying the activity of curcumin in these processes will be described below.

Role of Curcumin in Reducing Wound Inflammation

In addition to the aforementioned studies demonstrating the impact of curcumin on wound inflammation, extensive scientific research has documented anti-inflammatory effects of curcumin in a variety of inflammatory animal models, such as carrageenan-induced paw edema, experimentally induced ulcerative colitis, rheumatoid arthritis, pancreatitis, and cancer. Furthermore, in a clinical study conducted in patients with inguinal hernias or hydroceles post-surgery, curcumin and phenylbutazone (a type of non-steroidal anti-inflammatory drug) produced better anti-inflammatory responses in terms of spermatic cord edema/tenderness and operative site pain/tenderness than placebo [302].

In 2003, Chainani-Wu conducted a systematic review of the literature regarding the safety and anti-inflammatory activity of curcumin. The studies included *in vitro*, animal, and human studies. In six human trials, curcumin was found to be safe at doses of up to 8000 mg per day for three months in one trial and 1125-2500 mg per day in the other five trials. Laboratory studies have revealed that curcumin exerts anti-inflammatory activity by inhibiting a number of different molecules involved in inflammation, including phospholipase, LOX, COX-2, leukotrienes, thromboxane, prostaglandins, nitric oxide, collagenase, elastase, hyaluronidase, MCP-1, interferon-inducible protein, TNF, and IL-12 [303].

The following section describes the mechanisms underlying the anti-inflammatory properties of curcumin, based on investigations related to skin and wounds. As shown in Figure 11, the mechanisms implicated in the inhibitory effect of curcumin on wound inflammation could include the following: 1) suppression of the activities of inflammatory enzymes, such as COX, LOX, and MMPs; 2) inhibition of pro-inflammatory cytokine production; 3) stabilization of the lysosomal membrane; and 4) antioxidant activity.

Antithromboxane/Antiprostaglandin/Antileukotriene Activities

Curcumin has been shown to inhibit the biosynthesis of pro-inflammatory eicosanoids (thromboxanes, prostaglandins, and leukotrienes) from arachidonic acid through the COX and LOX enzymatic pathways. The topical application of curcumin significantly inhibited arachidonic acid-induced inflammation in mouse skin [304].

With reference to the COX pathway, *in vitro* studies have demonstrated that curcumin markedly reduces the arachidonic acid-induced production of prostaglandins (PGE2, PGF2-alpha, and PGD) by epidermal cells [304]. The production of thromboxanes (TXA2 and TXB2), the other eicosanoids derived from the COX pathway, were also inhibited by curcumin in *in vitro* studies in blood platelets [305, 306].

The inhibitory effect of curcumin on COX is due to its inhibition of COX-2 expression at the protein and mRNA levels, as well as of the catalytic activity of the enzyme [307]. Chun et al. demonstrated that enhanced expression of COX-2 in the mouse epidermis after phorbol ester induction was markedly suppressed by pretreatment with curcumin [308]. Kim et al. also showed that curcumin suppressed the mRNA expression of COX-2 but not that of COX-1 [309]. Further evidence indicated that this inhibition of COX-2 by curcumin was mediated by the suppression of extracellular signal-regulated kinase activity and by NF-κB activation [308].

The LOX pathway is also impeded by curcumin, thus suppressing pro-inflammatory leukotriene synthesis. Curcumin has been found to be a potent inhibitor of 5-hydroxy-eicosatetranoic acid (5-HETE) and 8-HETE production by epidermal cells [304] and of 5-HETE production by intact human neutrophils [310]. The down-regulation of LOX by curcumin occurs through direct inhibition of the enzyme activity of 5-LOX [307].

In addition to the inhibition of COX and LOX, which are enzymes involved in arachidonic acid metabolism, another mechanism underlying the inhibitory effects of curcumin on prostaglandin, thromboxane and leukotriene synthesis is its ability to prevent the incorporation of arachidonic acid into membrane phospholipids and to interfere with the liberation of arachidonic acid from phospholipids [305]. The latter is caused by a blockade of the phosphorylation of cytosolic phospholipase A2 enzyme, rather than direct inhibition of the activity of the enzyme [307].

Antihistamine Activity

The activity of histamine, one of the inflammatory vasoactive amines produced during inflammation, is diminished by curcumin. In addition to inhibiting eicosanoid production, curcumin has been shown to abrogate histamine release from mast cells activated by IgE or by the calcium ionophore A23187 [311, 312].

Inhibition of Inflammatory Cytokine and Enzyme Activity

Curcumin appears to modulate the inflammatory response, at least in part, by inhibiting the production of pro-inflammatory cytokines while activating anti-inflammatory cytokines. *In vivo*, Kant et al. showed that 25% and 0.3% of curcumin in a pluronic gel, applied topically on open excision skin wounds in a diabetic rat model, decreased the expression of inflammatory cytokines, including TNF-alpha and IL-1 beta, and the inflammatory enzyme MMP-9, which mediated leukocyte migration during inflammation. Simultaneously, curcumin increased the levels of the anti-inflammatory cytokine IL-10, as well as of antioxidant enzymes, including superoxide dismutase, catalase, and glutathione peroxidase [313]. Based on the experiment in human umbilical vein endothelial cells by Gupta et al., curcumin also blocked TNF-alpha-induced expression of the adhesion molecules ICAM-1, VCAM-1 and E-selectin, which play roles in leukocyte rolling and adhesion during the process of leukocyte recruitment to wound sites [314]. Using rabbit ear wound models under non-ischemic, ischemic, and ischemia reperfusion conditions to create normal and impaired healing conditions, the intravenous administration of curcumin improved healing, and this effect was associated with a decrease in the pro-inflammatory cytokines IL-1, IL-6, and IL-8 [315].

According to Murrell et al., curcumin nanofibers, which were developed to test the potential of curcumin as a wound dressing, reduced IL-6 production by mouse monocyte-macrophages following lipopolysaccharide-induced inflammation [316]. The inhibitory effects of curcumin on the production of other inflammatory cytokines, including IL-8, macrophage-inflammatory protein-1-alpha (MIP-1-alpha), and MCP-1, in addition to IL-1-beta, and TNF-alpha, by human peripheral blood monocytes and alveolar macrophages, as well as that of IL-12 in lipopolysaccharide-activated macrophages, have also been reported [317, 318].

Evidence from *in vitro* studies has suggested that curcumin attenuates inflammatory cytokine production through at least two principal mechanisms. First, it controls the activation of some nuclear factors, such as nuclear factor-kappa-B and activating protein-1 (AP-1), in stimulated monocytes and alveolar macrophages, subsequently blocking cytokine gene expression. Second, it down-regulates intercellular signaling proteins, such as protein kinase C, in mouse embryonic fibroblast cell lines [319-321].

Stabilization of the Lysosomal Membrane

One of the anti-inflammatory mechanisms of curcumin is lysosomal membrane stabilization. This effect was demonstrated by Joe and Lokesh, who revealed that curcumin could reduce the release of lysosomal enzymes from activated macrophages [322]. The suppression of lysosomal enzymes, which are inflammatory mediators, subsequently reduces the inflammatory response.

Antioxidant Activity

It is well established that curcumin is a powerful antioxidant and superoxide scavenger [323]. It can inhibit lipid peroxidation and reduce reactive oxygen species production, as well as increase the levels of antioxidant enzymes, including superoxide dismutase, catalase, and glutathione peroxidase, in wound tissues [313, 324].

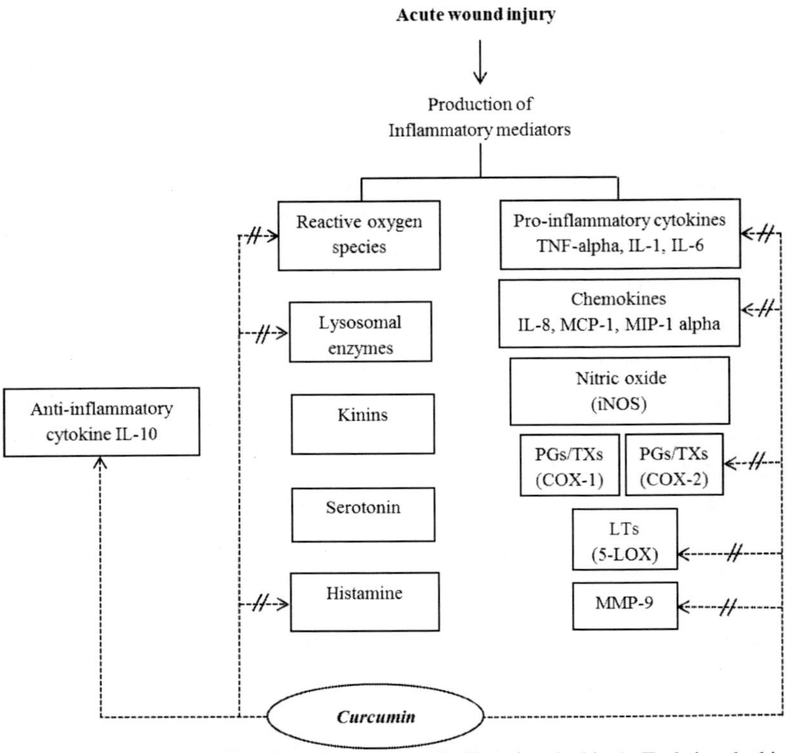

COX-1, cyclooxygenase-1; COX-2, cyclooxygenase-2; IL-1, interleukin-1; IL-6, interleukin-6; IL-8, interleukin-8; iNOS, inducible nitric oxide synthase; 5-LOX, 5-lipoxygenase; LTs, leukotrienes; MCP-1, monocyte chemoattractant protein-1; MIP-1 alpha, macrophage-inflammatory protein-1 alpha; MMP-9, matrix metalloproteinase-9; PGs, prostaglandins; TNF-alpha, tumor necrosis factor-alpha; TXs, thromboxanes.

Figure 11. Inhibition by curcumin, an active substance in *Curcuma longa,* of the inflammatory mediators that are produced during wound inflammation. Curcumin reduces the expression of inflammatory cytokines by inhibiting the activation of certain nuclear factors, such as nuclear factor-kappa-B and activating protein-1. Curcumin also increases the levels of the anti-inflammatory cytokine IL-10. Enzymes that stimulate the synthesis of NO, PGs/TXs, and LTs are shown in parentheses.

Role of Curcumin in Wound Angiogenesis

It was mentioned previously that curcumin helps to heal wounds by increasing angiogenesis [283, 288-291]. Although several studies have shown that curcumin is an inhibitor of cancer-associated angiogenesis [325-328], Kiran et al. suggested that curcumin exhibits pro-angiogenic activity in the absence of extracellular stimuli derived from serum [329].

Kiran et al. found that, when cells were treated with curcumin under serum-free conditions, there was an increment of sprouting in the rat aortic ring, vascular density in the chorio-allantoic membrane, and morphological changes suggestive of an angiogenic phenotype in human umbilical vein endothelial cells and rat aortic endothelial cells in culture. The expression of angiogenic biochemical markers also increased. These effects were dependent on VEGF, which was mediated through activation of the PI3K-Akt pathway. Contrasting effects were observed under serum-stimulated conditions in which curcumin inhibited the MAPK pathway.

These findings indicated that curcumin might cause different angiogenic responses, depending on the extracellular microenvironment [329].

Role of Curcumin in Matrix Formation and Remodeling

As previously described, curcumin can improve cell proliferation, matrix deposition and remodeling in both normal and impaired healing models. Additionally, the treatment of rabbit ear wounds under non-ischemic, ischemic, and ischemia reperfusion conditions with intravenous curcumin improved healing in terms of re-epithelialization and granulation tissue formation [315]. An example of a study demonstrating the efficacy of curcumin on the proliferative and remodeling phases of wound healing is that conducted by Panchatcharam et al., using a full-thickness excision wound model in rats. Topical curcumin resulted in enhanced cellular proliferation (as evidenced by an increase in DNA and total protein), type III collagen synthesis, epithelialization rates, and wound contraction. There were also increases in the stability of acid-soluble collagen, aldehyde content, shrinkage temperature and tensile strength, indicating improved maturation and crosslinking of collagen during wound remodeling [324]. Mohanty et al. stated that accelerated wound healing by curcumin could be ascribed to the early deposition of fibroblasts and their differentiation, as gauged by increased levels of alpha-smooth muscle actin [296].

Based on the available evidence, the positive roles of curcumin in matrix formation, re-epithelialization, and tissue remodeling occur at both the cellular and molecular levels. At the cellular level, curcumin has been shown to possess free radical-scavenging activity, which aids in protecting keratinocytes and fibroblasts against oxidative damage. At the molecular level, curcumin acts through two mechanisms: the regulation of TGF-beta and the modulation of urokinase plasminogen activator (uPA) expression.

A number of studies have demonstrated the wound healing properties of curcumin from an antioxidant perspective. By virtue of its ability to quench reactive oxygen species, curcumin protects skin cells. Phan et al. showed that curcumin at doses of 2.5 and 10 mcg/mL had significant inhibitory effects on hydrogen peroxide-induced damage to cultured human keratinocytes and fibroblasts [330]. Curcumin-loaded poly(epsilon-caprolactone) nanofibers not only have wound healing capabilities and reduce pro-inflammatory cytokines *in vivo,* as described previously, but they also maintained the viability of human foreskin fibroblasts by more than 70% under oxidative stress conditions *in vitro* [316]. Panchatcharam et al. showed that curcumin treatment of full-thickness excision wounds in rats resulted in a decrease in lipid peroxides while increasing the activity levels of antioxidant enzymes, including superoxide dismutase, catalase, and glutathione peroxidase [324]. Singer et al. showed that burn injury progression, owing in part to “highly reactive oxygen radicals”, was reduced by the antioxidant activity of curcumin and that this effect was not mediated by iron chelation, which is the process of iron removal that induces the formation of reactive oxygen species (hydrogen peroxide and superoxide) and converts them into highly reactive oxygen species [285, 286]. Similarly, impaired diabetic wound healing, which is characterized by prolonged inflammation and increased oxidative stress, is improved by curcumin through both its anti-inflammatory and antioxidant potential. Kant et al. reported that the topical application of curcumin (0.3% and 25% in pluronic gel) could accelerate the repair of excision skin wounds in streptozotocin-induced diabetic rats, as well as increase the levels of antioxidant enzymes, including superoxide dismutase, catalase, and glutathione peroxidase, in wound tissues [313].

In terms of the molecular mechanisms underlying the effects of curcumin on ECM formation and tissue remodeling, *in vivo* studies have indicated that curcumin enhances TGF-beta 1, one of the most important peptide growth factors involved in the wound healing process. Sidhu et al. demonstrated an increase in TGF-beta-1, as well as mRNA transcripts of TGF-beta-1 and fibronectin, in the curcumin-treated punch wounds of normal rats and guinea pigs [283]. Similarly, in diabetic impaired healing, oral and topical curcumin facilitated wound repair, concurrent with elevations of TGF-beta-1 and TGF-beta-1 mRNA expression in wound tissues [287]. However, curcumin seemed to exert differential regulatory effects on TGF-beta 1, its receptors, and inducible nitric oxide synthase (iNOS) in comparisons of normal and impaired wound healing. Mani et al. reported that curcumin enhanced the expression of TGF-beta-1 and TGF-beta receptor type II, as well as TGF-beta-1 mRNA expression in macrophages in the wound beds of both normal and dexamethasone-impaired healing wounds. However, curcumin was able to enhance TGF-beta receptor type I expression only in dexamethasone-impaired healing wounds and to increase levels of iNOS only in normal wounds [331].

The second molecular mechanism of curcumin is its modulation of urokinase plasminogen activator (uPA) expression, which provides the proteolytic potential that promotes fibrin dissolution and cellular migration to wound sites [332]. It has been proposed that the up-regulation of uPA by curcumin is mediated by the activation of JNK and p38 mitogen-activated protein kinase (MAPK) signaling pathways. Although research has shown that curcumin does not induce fibroblast migration kinematics *in vitro* [183], it is likely that curcumin indirectly facilitates fibroblast migration during wound healing *in vivo* by increasing fibrin dissolution, which facilitates the movement of fibroblasts into the wound bed.

Role of Curcumin in the Modulation of Scar Formation

Evidence has indicated that a high concentration of curcumin could potentially reduce pathological scar formation by inducing fibroblast apoptosis and inhibiting the growth and function of fibroblasts. Scharstuhl et al. noted that low-dose curcumin (5 mcmol/L) provided protection against fibroblast apoptosis, whereas high-dose curcumin of at least 25 mcmol/L increased fibroblast apoptosis and also prevented fibroblast-mediated collagen gel contraction in an *in vitro* wound contraction model [333].

In another study, Kang et al. found that curcumin tended to inhibit growth and collagen type I synthesis in fibroblasts derived from human hypertrophic scar tissue at doses of 25-100 mcmol/L, with significant effects at doses of 50 and 100 mcmol/L [334]. The intravenous administration of purified curcumin reduced hypertrophic scarring in rabbit ear models of non-ischemic, ischemic, and ischemia-reperfusion wounds [315].

Given that fibroblast apoptosis and the inhibition of over-exuberant wound contraction contribute to the reduction of pathological scar formation, the above findings should expedite more detailed explorations of the anti-scarring effect of curcumin.

Role of Curcumin As an Antimicrobial Agent

Curcumin has been shown to exhibit antibacterial, antifungal, and antiviral activities. *In vitro* studies have shown that curcumin is active against strains of *S. aureus* and *C. albicans,* both of which are common causes of wound infections [335, 336]. Other microorganisms that are susceptible to curcumin include *Salmonella paratyphi, Trichophyton gypseum, M. tuberculosis,* Herpes simplex virus-1, and Coxsackie virus [335, 337, 338]. In accordance with a very recent study by Krausz et al., curcumin-encapsulated nanoparticles inhibited the *in vitro* growth of methicillin-resistant *S. aureus* and *P. auruginosa* in a dose-dependent manner. A parallel *in vivo* experiment in a murine burn wound model also demonstrated the effects of curcumin-encapsulated nanoparticles on the inhibition of the growth of methicillin-resistant *S. aureus* and on the enhancement of wound healing [339].

Conclusion

The mechanisms of action of *Aloe vera, Centella asiatica,* and *Curcuma longa* are summarized in Table 3. These herbal medicines share some commonalities. The three medicinal plants contribute to every key component of the wound healing process, leading to an acceleration of wound healing by virtue of their diverse biological activities; however, certain herbs have prominent capabilities or mechanisms.

1 They have anti-inflammatory activity that is arbitrated by the inhibition of inflammatory mediators, such as prostaglandins, thromboxanes, leukotrienes, histamine, and bradykinin. They also reduce the levels of pro-inflammatory cytokines and enzymes, as well as of the free radicals generated during the inflammatory phase of wound healing. These reductions result in the early resolution of inflammation, which could aid in reducing scar development, diminishing tissue damage and providing pain relief. In particular, these anti-inflammatory effects can ameliorate the delayed or impaired wound healing observed in diabetic or irradiated wounds caused by prolonged and excessive inflammation. The molecular mechanism by which *Centella asiatica* and *Curcuma longa* inhibit COX and pro-inflammatory cytokines has been shown to occur

largely through NF-κB inactivation, but that of *Aloe vera* remains to be elucidated by further investigations.

2 As antioxidant agents, the three herbal medicines not only help to suppress wound inflammation, but they also protect against oxidative damage various cells that are involved in the healing process, such as fibroblasts and keratinocytes, which play critical roles in collagen synthesis and re-epithelialization, respectively.

3 Unlike other anti-inflammatory agents, such as NSAIDs or steroids, which impair angiogenesis and retard the healing process by interrupting the balance between prostaglandins and TXA2 [340], these herbals, despite having anti-inflammatory properties, can enhance angiogenesis and promote tissue repair and remodeling. For *Aloe vera*, this characteristic might be due to the presence of a large combination of active compounds that act in concert to modulate the response, with glycoproteins and acemannan (or mannose-6-phosphate) functioning as the main compounds responsible for its anti-inflammatory and wound healing effects, respectively. *Aloe vera* works by activating the growth factors and enzymes that are involved in the proliferative and remodeling stages of wound healing, such as TGF-beta-1, VEGF, KGF-1, and bFGF. For *Centella asiatica*, asiatic acid and madecassic acid have been examined for their anti-inflammatory activities, while asiaticoside and madecassoside are effective in activating angiogenesis and in promoting collagen synthesis and re-epithelialization through the TGF-beta/Smad pathway. For *Curcuma longa*, curcumin might be the one compound that has received a large amount of attention and that has pleiotropic effects due to its ability to act via many signaling pathways. These pathways include the PI3K-Akt pathway for angiogenesis and the TGF-beta pathway, as well as JNK and p38 MAPK signaling pathways for matrix formation and remodeling. The cellular and molecular mechanisms of *Aloe vera* in wound re-epithelialization are better understood than those provided by *Centella asiatica* and *Curcuma longa,* which remain to be elucidated. To standardize the assessment of wound healing progression, it is suggested that *in vivo* animal experiments should consider using a quantification system for the analysis of each stage-specific parameter, similar to the method described by Braiman-Wiksman et al. [341].

4 In addition to their direct effects on the healing process, the three herbal medicines also play roles in modifying factors that influence

wound healing, which are among the wound management strategies. Interestingly, these herbal medicines possess antimicrobial activity, which aids in preventing and controlling wound infection. Moreover, *Aloe vera* has been shown to promote oxygenation, vascularization, and moisturization, providing a local wound environment for optimal healing. Microcirculatory studies using an intravital microscopy technique have provided beautiful results for the *in vivo* vascularization effect of *Aloe vera*, and such studies are needed to affirm this effect for *Centella asiatica* and *Curcuma longa.*

5 The role for herbal medicine in scar management is another facet of interest. Among the three medicinal plants, *Centella asiatica* appears to have been investigated extensively for its effect on scar prevention and for the management of hypertrophic and keloid scars. Asiaticoside has been shown to inhibit type I collagen expression, suppress TGF-beta/Smad signaling, down-regulate TGF-beta 1 mRNA and TIMP 1 expression and up-regulate TGF-beta 3 expression in hypertrophic and keloid scars, in opposition to its effects on normal wounds. Asiatic acid inhibits collagen type I and PAI-1 expression, as well as Smad 2/3 phosphorylation, while elevating Smad 7 protein levels via PPAR-gamma activation. Madecassoside suppresses the migration of keloid-derived fibroblasts via the p38 kinase and PI3K signaling pathways.

6 Systematic reviews documenting clinical efficacy in skin wound healing are only available for *Aloe vera,* which is potentially effective in the treatment of first and second degree burns. Its clinical effectiveness, however, remains inconclusive. There remains a need for well-designed, randomized, controlled trials with high methodological quality, valid wound healing assessment strategies and standardization of the herbal products. Additionally, the efficacy of using the active ingredients of these medicinal plants in wound healing dressings and drug delivery systems is a fruitful area of exploration.

In conclusion, *Aloe vera, Centella asiatica, and Curcuma longa* can facilitate cutaneous wound healing and repair by suppressing inflammation, promoting angiogenesis, inducing cellular growth and proliferation, reducing wound oxidative stress, controlling infection, and improving wound remodeling.

This chapter has provided the possible explanations and mechanisms for how these herbal medicines and their responsible active ingredients exert their effects at biochemical, cellular, and molecular levels. A better understanding of the basic therapeutic mechanisms will facilitate future research supporting the development of newer and more effective nature-derived formulations for cutaneous wound care.

Table 3. Mechanisms of action of *Aloe vera, Centella asiatica, and Curcuma longa* in each key component of the wound healing process

Suppression of wound inflammation		
Aloe vera	*Centella asiatica*	*Curcuma longa*
a. Antithromboxane/antiprostaglandin activities		
- inhibits arachidonic acid oxidation - inhibits arachidonic acid release from phospholipids by inhibiting phospholipase A2 - inhibits COX enzyme activity - inhibits COX-2 and TXA2 synthase	- inhibits COX-2 expression through NF-κB inactivation - suppresses both COX-1 and COX-2 activities	- inhibits the incorporation of arachidonic acid into membrane phospholipids - interferes with the liberation of arachidonic acid from phospholipids - inhibits the mRNA and protein expression of COX-2 via suppression of extracellular signal-regulated kinase activity and NF-κB activation
b. Antileukotriene activity		
- inhibits mass 1,2-diacylglycerol formation and phospholipase activity	Data not available	- directly inhibits the enzyme activity of 5-LOX - inhibits the incorporation of arachidonic acid into membrane phospholipids - interferes with the liberation of arachidonic acid from phospholipids by blocking the phosphorylation of cytosolic phospholipase A2 enzyme, rather than by directly inhibiting the enzyme activity

Table 3. (Continued)

Suppression of wound inflammation		
Aloe vera	*Centella asiatica*	*Curcuma longa*
c. Antibradykinin activity		
- hydrolyzes bradykinin	- inhibits the liberation of kinins	Data not available
d. Antihistamine activity		
- inhibits the conversion of histidine into histamine in mast cells by inhibiting histidine decarboxylase - inhibits histamine release from mast cells	- inhibits histamine release from mast cells	- inhibits histamine release from mast cells
e. Inhibition of pro-inflammatory cytokines/enzymes		
- decreases serum levels of TNF-alpha and IL-6 - inhibits MMP-9	- inhibits the expression of the pro-inflammatory cytokines IL-6, IL-1 beta, and TNF-alpha via NF-κB inactivation - stimulates TNF and AIP6 expression	- inhibits TNF-alpha, IL-1beta, IL-1, IL-6, IL-8, and IL-12 - inhibits MMP-9, MIP-1 alpha, and MCP-1 - increases the anti-inflammatory cytokine IL-10 - blocks cytokine gene expression by inhibiting NF-κB and AP-1 activation
f. Other anti-inflammatory activities		
- antioxidant activity - inhibits the degradation of vascular basement membrane ECM by inhibiting lysosomal enzyme-mannose phosphate receptor interaction	- antioxidant activity - stabilizes the lysosomal membrane	- antioxidant activity - stabilizes the lysosomal membrane
Enhancement of wound angiogenesis		
Aloe vera	*Centella asiatica*	*Curcuma longa*
- activates the expression of proteins involved in angiogenesis, such as TGF-beta-1, VEGF, VEGF-R2 or Flk-1, von Willebrand factor, and blood vessel matrix laminin	- enhances the expression of genes encoding pro-angiogenic factors, such as PAI-2, VEGF, FGF-1, and FGF-2	- increases VEGF through activation of the PI3K-Akt pathway under serum-free conditions

Enhancement of wound angiogenesis		
Aloe vera	*Centella asiatica*	*Curcuma longa*
- stimulates the production of TGF-beta and basic FGF (bFGF or FGF-2) - enhances the expression of u-PA, MMP-2, and MT-MMP - stimulates endothelial cell migration	- reduces the expression of anti-angiogenic thrombospondin - increases the expression of MCP-1 and IL-1-beta, which enhance VEGF production	- increases VEGF through activation of the PI3K-Akt pathway under serum-free conditions
Promotion of matrix formation and remodeling		
Aloe vera	*Centella asiatica*	*Curcuma longa*
- stimulates fibroblast proliferation and collagen synthesis, with no effect on fibroblast migration - increases KGF-1 and bFGF expression - binds to FGF-2 receptors or affects the FGF-2 signaling pathway - inhibits the activity of granulocyte MMPs, most likely by destabilizing the enzyme structure - enhances MMP-3 and TIMP-2 gene expression	- induces the migration, initial adhesion, and proliferation of normal human skin fibroblasts - up-regulates the expression of genes encoding cell proliferation and cell-cycle progression in fibroblasts - increases the expression of hyaladherin and cytokines, including PAI-2 and TGF-beta - activates the TGF-beta/Smad pathway - increases the mRNA expression of TGF-beta receptor II and the phosphorylation of Smad 3 and elevates TGF-beta 1 levels	- protects fibroblasts against oxidative damage through free radical scavenging activity - enhances the expression of TGF-beta-1 and TGF-beta receptor type II, as well as TGF-beta-1 mRNA, in both normal and dexamethasone-impaired healing wounds, but enhances TGF-beta receptor type I expression only in dexamethasone-impaired healing wounds - does not directly induce fibroblast migration but indirectly facilitates fibroblast migration by increasing fibrin dissolution through the upregulation of uPA via activation of JNK and p38 MAPK signaling pathways
Acceleration of wound re-epithelialization		
Aloe vera	*Centella asiatica*	*Curcuma longa*
- accelerates the proliferation and migration of human keratinocytes	- stimulates the cells of the Malphigian layer and activates keratinization	- protects keratinocytes against oxidative damage through free radical scavenging activity

Table 3. (Continued)

Acceleration of wound re-epithelialization		
Aloe vera	*Centella asiatica*	*Curcuma longa*
- increases the expression of proliferation markers, including epidermal growth factor receptor, fibronectin receptor, fibronectin, keratin 5/14 and keratin 1/10 - increases the expression of KGF and FGF-2, which regulate the migration and proliferation of keratinocytes	- increases the migration and initial adhesion, but not the proliferation, of the keratinocytes of the epidermal layers	- protects keratinocytes against oxidative damage through free radical scavenging activity
Improvement of keloids and hypertrophic scars		
Aloe vera	*Centella asiatica*	*Curcuma longa*
Data not available	- inhibits inflammation, decreases collagen synthesis, increases collagen degradation, and promotes scar maturity <u>Asiaticoside</u> - inhibits type I and type II collagen expression and TGF-beta/Smad signaling via induction of Smad7 and suppression of TGF-beta receptor-1 and TGF-beta receptor-2, with no effects on Smad2 - down-regulates TGF-beta-1 mRNA and TIMP-1 expression and up-regulates TGF-beta-3 expression; MMP expression not affected <u>Asiatic acid</u> - inhibits collagen type I and PAI-1 expression	- reduces pathological scar formation via a high concentration of curcumin, which induces fibroblast apoptosis and inhibits the growth and function of fibroblasts

Improvement of keloids and hypertrophic scars		
Aloe vera	*Centella asiatica*	*Curcuma longa*
Data not available	- inhibits Smad 2/3 phosphorylation while elevating Smad 7 protein levels via PPAR-gamma activation Madecassoside - suppresses the migration of keloid-derived fibroblasts via the p38 kinase and PI3K signaling pathways	- reduces pathological scar formation via a high concentration of curcumin, which induces fibroblast apoptosis and inhibits the growth and function of fibroblasts
Modification of factors that affect wound healing		
Aloe vera	*Centella asiatica*	*Curcuma longa*
- antimicrobial activity - promotes oxygenation and vascularization by restoring endothelial function and stimulating angiogenesis - provides moisturization of wounds via the high water content of aloe gel - provides a source of nutrition, including polysaccharides, amino acids, vitamins (vitamin A, C, and E), and minerals (zinc, copper, iron and magnesium)	- antimicrobial activity	- antimicrobial activity

AP-1, activating protein-1; COX-1, COX-2, cyclooxygenases-1 and -2; ECM, extracellular matrix; FGF-1, FGF-2, fibroblast growth factors-1 and -2; Flk-1, fetal liver kinase-1; IL-1, IL-1 beta, IL-6, IL-8, IL-10, IL-12, interleukins-1, -1 beta, -6, -8, -10, and -12; JNK, c-Jun N-terminal kinase; KGF-1, keratinocyte growth factor-1; 5-LOX, 5-lipoxygenase; MAPK, mitogen-activated protein kinases; MCP-1, monocyte chemoattractant protein-1; MIP-1 alpha, monocyte (or macrophage)-inflammatory protein-1 alpha; MMP-2, MMP-3, MMP-9, matrix metalloproteinases-2, -3 and -9; MT-MMP, membrane-type matrix metalloproteinase; NF-κB, nuclear factor-kappa-B; PAI-2, plasminogen activator inhibitor-2; PI3K-Akt, phosphoinositide-3-kinase–Akt; TGF-beta-1, transforming growth factor-beta-1; TIMP-2, tissue inhibitor of matrix metalloproteinase-2; TNF-alpha, tumor necrosis factor-alpha; TXA2, thromboxane A2; u-PA, urokinase-type plasminogen activator; VEGF, vascular endothelial growth factor; VEGF-R2, vascular endothelial growth factor receptor 2.

References

[1] Enoch, S., Leaper, D. J. Basic science of wound healing. *Surgery*, 2007, 26, 31-7.

[2] Kumar, V., Abbas, A. K., Aster, J. C. *Robbins Basic Pathology*. 9th edition. Philadelphia, PA: Elsevier Saunders; 2013.

[3] Sephel, G., Davidson, J. M. Repair, regeneration and fibrosis. In: Rubin E, Reisner HM, editors. *Essentials of Rubin's Pathology*. 6th edition. Philadelphia, PA: Lippincott Williams and Wilkins; 2014; 49-69.

[4] Edwards, R., Harding, K. G. Bacteria and wound healing. *Curr. Opin. Infect. Dis.*, 2004, 17, 91-6.

[5] Davis, S. C., Ricotti, C., Cazzanica, A., Welsh, E., Eaglstein, W. H., Mertz, P. M. Microscopic and physiologic evidence for biofilm-associated wound colonization *in vivo*. *Wound Repair. Regen.*, 2008, 16, 23-9.

[6] Bishop, A. Role of oxygen in wound healing. *J. Wound Care,* 2008, 17, 399-402.

[7] Knighton, D. R., Hunt, T. K., Scheuenstuhl, H., Halliday, B. J., Werb, Z., Banda, M. J. Oxygen tension regulates the expression of angiogenesis factor by macrophages. *Science*, 1983, 221, 1283-5.

[8] Gottrup, F. Oxygen in wound healing and infection. *World J. Surg*., 2004, 28, 312-5.

[9] Räkel, A., Huot, C., Ekoé, J. M. Canadian Diabetes Association technical review: The diabetic foot and hyperbaric oxygen therapy. *Can. J. Diabetes*, 2006, 30, 411-21.

[10] Stone, A. J., Cianci, P. The adjunctive role of hyperbaric oxygen therapy in the treatment of lower extremity wounds in patients with diabetes. *Diabetes Spectrum*, 1997, 10, 118-23.

[11] Marston, W. Mixed arterial and venous ulcers. *Wounds,* 2011, 23, 351-6.

[12] Rovee, D. T., Kurowsky, C. A., Labun, J. Local wound environment and epidermal healing: mitotic response. *Arch. Dermatol.,* 1972, 106, 330-4.

[13] Hinman, C. D., Maibach, H. Effect of air exposure and occlusion on experimental human skin wounds. *Nature*, 1963, 200, 377-8.

[14] Knighton, D. R., Silver, J. A., Hunt, T. Regulation of wound healing angiogenesis: effect of oxygen gradients and inspired oxygen concentration. *Surgery*, 1981, 90, 262-70.

[15] Baxter, C. R. Immunologic reactions in chronic wounds. *Am. J. Surg*., 1994, 167, 12S-14S.

[16] Haimowitz, J. E., Margolis, J. Moist wound healing. In: Krasner, D., Kane, D., editors. *Chronic Wound Care: A Clinical Source Book for Healthcare Professionals*. Wayne, PA: Health Management Publications; 1997; 49-55.

[17] Mertz, P. M., Marshall, D. A., Eaglstein, W. H. Occlusive dressings to prevent bacterial invasion and wound infection. *J. Am. Acad. Dermatol.*, 1985, 12, 662-8.

[18] Harris, D. R. Healing of the surgical wound: II. Factors affecting repair and regeneration. *J. Am. Acad. Dermatol.*, 1979, 1, 208-15.

[19] Gosain, A., DiPietro, L. A. Aging and wound healing. *World J. Surg.*, 2004, 28, 321-6.

[20] Gilliver, S. C., Ashworth, J. J., Ashcroft, G. S. The hormonal regulation of cutaneous wound healing. *Clin. Dermatol.*, 2007, 25, 56-62.

[21] Hardman, M. J., Ashcroft, G. S. Estrogen, not intrinsic aging, is the major regulator of delayed human wound healing in the elderly. *Genome Biol.,* 2008, 9, R80.

[22] Shepherd, A. A. Nutrition for optimal wound healing. *Nurs. Stand.*, 2003, 18, 55-8.

[23] Breslow, R. A., Hallfrisch, J., Guy, D. G., Crawley, B., Goldberg, A. P. The importance of dietary protein in healing pressure ulcers. *J. Am. Geriatr. Soc.*, 1993, 41, 357-62.

[24] Daly, J. M., Reynolds, J., Sigal, R. K., Shou, J., Lieberman, M. D. Effect of dietary protein and amino acids in the immune system. *Crit. Care Med.*, 1990, 18, 86-93.

[25] Tong, B. C., Barbul, A. Cellular ad physiological effects of arginine. *Mini Rev. Med. Chem.*, 2004, 4, 823-32.

[26] Witte, M. B., Barbul, A. Role of nitric oxide in wound repair. *Am. J. Surg.*, 2002, 183, 406-12.

[27] Arnold, M., Barbul, A. Nutrition and wound healing. *Plast. Reconstr. Surg.*, 2006, 117, 42S-58S.

[28] da Costa, M. A., Campos, A. C., Coelho, J. C., de Barros, A. M., Matsumoto, H. M. Oral glutamine and the healing of colonic anastomoses in rats. *J. Parenter. Enteral Nutr.,* 2003, 27,182-5.

[29] Senel, O., Cetinkale, O., Ozbay, G., Ahçioğlu, F., Bulan, R. Oxygen free radicals impair wound healing in ischemic rat skin. *Ann. Plast. Surg.*, 1997, 39, .23-516

[30] Burns, J. L., Mancoll, J. S., Phillips, L. G. Impairments to wound healing .*Clin. Plast. Surg.*, 2003, 30, .56-47

[31] Weinzweig, J., Levenson, S. M., Rettura, G., Weinzweig, N., Mendecki, J., Chang, T. H., Seifter, E. Supplemental vitamin A prevents the tumor-induced defect in wound healing. *Ann. Surg.*,1990 , 211, 269-.76

[32] Ross, A. C. Vitamin A and protective immunity. *Nutr. Today*, 1992, 27, 18-26.

[33] Burgess, C. Topical vitamins. *J. Drugs Dermatol.*, 2008, 7, s2-s6.

[34] Lawrence, D. J., Bern, H. A., Steadman, M. G. Vitamin A and keratinization .Studies on the hamster cheekpouch. *Ann. Otol. Rhinol. Laryngol.,* 1960, 69, 645-60.

[35] Khoosal, D., Goldman, R. D. Vitamin E for treating children's scars. Does it help reduce scarring? *Can. Fam. Physician*,2006 , 52, .6-855

[36] Ehrlich, H. P., Hunt, T. K. The effects of cortisone and anabolic steroids on the tensile strength of healing wounds. *Ann. Surg*.,1969 ,170 , 203-.6

[37] Boyapati, L., Wang, H. L. The role of stress in periodontal disease and wound healing. *Periodontol.* 2000, 2007, 44, 195-210.

[38] Wilson, J. A., Clark, J. J. Obesity: impediment to postsurgical wound healing. *Adv. Skin Wound Care*, 2004, 17, 426-35.

[39] Juge-Aubry, C. E., Henrichot, E., Meier, C. A. Adipose tissue: a regulator of inflammation. *Best Pract. Res. Clin. Endocrinol. Metab*., 2005, 19, 547-66.

[40] Calabro, P., Yeh, E. T. Obesity, inflammation, and vascular disease: the role of the adipose tissue as an endocrine gland. *Subcell. Biochem*., 2007, 42, 63-91.

[41] Choudhry, M. A., Chaudry, I. H. Alcohol intoxication and post-burn complications. *Front. Biosci.*, 2006, 11, 998-1005.

[42] Radek, K. A., Matthies, A. M., Burns, A. L., Heinrich, S. A., Kovacs, E. J., Dipietro, L. A. Acute ethanol exposure impairs angiogenesis and the proliferative phase of wound healing. *Am. J. Physiol. Heart Circ. Physiol.*, 2005, 289, H1084-90.

[43] Chan, L. K., Withey, S., Butler, P. E. Smoking and wound healing problems in reduction mammaplasty: is the introduction of urine nicotine testing justified? *Ann. Plast. Surg*., 2006, 56, 111-5.

[44] Ahn, C., Mulligan, P., Salcido, R. S. Smoking – the bane of wound healing: biomedical interventions and social. *Adv. Skin Wound Care*, 2008, 21, 227-38.

[45] Franz, M. G., Steed, D. L., Robson, M. C. Optimizing healing of the acute wound by minimizing complications. *Curr. Probl. Surg*., 2007, 44, 691-763.

[46] Hofman, D., Moore, K., Eagle, M., Cooper, S. Use of topical corticosteroids on chronic leg ulcers. *J. Wound Care*, 2007, 16, 227-30.

[47] Dvivedi, S., Tiwari, S. M., Sharma, A. Effect of ibuprofen and diclofenac sodium on experimental wound healing. *Indian J. Exp. Biol.*, 1997, 35, 1243-5.

[48] Loots, M. A., Lamme, E. N., Zeegelaar, J., Mekkes, J. R., Bos, J. D., Middelkoop, E. Differences in cellular infiltrate and extracellular matrix of chronic diabetic and venous ulcers versus acute wounds. *J. Invest. Dermatol.*, 1998, 111, 850-7.

[49] Guo, S., DiPietro, L. A. Factors affecting wound healing. *J. Dent. Res.*, 2010, 89, 219-29.

[50] Tandara, A. A., Mustoe, T. A. Oxygen in wound healing – more than a nutrient. *World J. Surg.*, 2004, 28, 294-300.

[51] Gallagher, K. A., Liu, Z. J., Xiao, M., Chen, H., Goldstein, L. J., Buerk, D. G., Nedeau, A., Thom, S. R., Velazquez, O. C. Diabetic impairments in NO-mediated endothelial progenitor cell mobilization and homing are reversed by hyperoxia and SDF-1 alpha. *J. Clin. Invest.*, 2007, 117, 1249-59.

[52] Woo, K., Ayello, E. A., Sibbald, R. G. The edge effect: current therapeutic options to advance the wound edge. *Adv. Skin Wound Care*, 2007, 20, 99-117.

[53] Vincent, A. M., Russell, J. W., Low, P., Feldman, E. L. Oxidative stress in the pathogenesis of diabetic neuropathy. *Endocr. Rev.*, 2004, 25, 612-28.

[54] Huijberts, M. S., Schaper, N. C., Schalkwijk, C. G. Advanced glycation end products and diabetic foot disease. *Diabetes Metab. Res. Rev.*, 2008, 24, S19-S24.

[55] Galkowska, H., Olszewski, W. L., Wojewodzka, U., Rosinski, G., Karnafel, W. Neurogenic factors in the impaired healing of diabetic foot ulcers. *J. Surg. Res.*, 2006, 134, 252-8.

[56] Canadian Association of Wound Care (CAWC). *CAWC Institute for Wound Management and Prevention, Level 1 Workbook: Putting Knowledge into Practice – Knowledge Learning.* Toronto: Canadian Association of Wound Care; 2010.

[57] Australian Wound Management Association. *Standard for Wound Management.* 2nd edition. West Leederville WA: Cambridge Publishing; 2010.

[58] Naude, L. The practice and science of wound healing: wound bed preparation utilising the guidelines. *Prof. Nurs. Today*, 2011, 15, 22-30.

[59] Sibbald, R. G., Orsted, H. L., Coutts, P. M., Keast, D. H. Best practice recommendations for preparing the wound bed: update 2006. *Wound Care Canada*, 2006, 4, 15-29.

[60] Jones, V., Grey, J. E., Harding, K. G. ABC of wound healing: wound dressings. *BMJ*, 2006, 332, 777-80.

[61] Flanagan, M. Improving accuracy of wound measurement in clinical practice. *Ostomy Wound Manage.*, 2003, 49, 28-40.

[62] Sullivan, T. P., Eaglstein, W. H., Davis, S. C., Mertz, P. The pig as a model for human wound healing. *Wound Repair Regen.,* 2001, 9, 66-76.

[63] Ansell, D. M., Holden, K. A., Hardman, M. J. Animal models of wound repair: Are they cutting it? *Exp. Dermatol.*, 2012, 21, 581-5.

[64] Mogford, J. E., Mustoe, T. A. Experimental models of wound healing. In: Falanga, V., editor. *Cutaneous Wound Healing.* London: Martin Dunitz Ltd.; 2001; 109-22.

[65] Galiano, R. D., Michaels, J., Dobryansky, M., Levine, J. P., Gurtner, G. C. Quantitative and reproducible murine model of excisional wound healing. *Wound Repair Regen.,* 2004, 12, 485-92.

[66] Dunn, L., Prosser, H. C. G., Tan, J. T. M., Vanags, L. Z., Ng, M. K. C., Bursill, C. A. Murine model of wound healing. *J. Vis. Exp.,* 2013, (75), e50265, doi:10.3791/50265.

[67] Naeini, A. T., Oryan, A., Dehghani, S., Nikahval, B. Experimental cutaneous wound healing in rabbits :using continuous microamperage low-voltage electrical stimulation. *Comp. Clin. Path.*, 2008, 17, 203-10.

[68] Dzubow, L. M., Miller, W. H., Jr. The effect of 13-cis-retinoic acid on wound healing in dogs. *J. Dermatol. Surg. Oncol.*, 1987, 13, 265-8.

[69] Swindle, M. M., Makin, A., Herron, A. J., Clubb, Jr, F. J., Frazier, K. S. Swine as models in biomedical research and toxicology testing. *Vet. Pathol.,* 2012, 49, 344-56.

[70] Keswani, S. G., Katz, A. B., Lim, F. Y., Zoltick, P., Radu, A., Alaee, D., Herlyn, M., Crombleholme, T. M. Adenoviral mediated gene transfer of PDGF-B enhances wound healing in type I and type II diabetic wounds. *Wound Repair Regen.*, 2004, 12, 497-504.

[71] Huang, Z., Lu, M., Zhu, G., Gao, H., Xie, L., Zhang, X., Ye, C., Wang, Y., Sun, C., Li, X. Acceleration of diabetic-wound healing with PEGylated rhaFGF in healing-impaired streptozocin diabetic rats. *Wound Repair Regen.,* 2011, 19, 633-44.

[72] Boquist, L., Hellman, B., Lernmark, A., Täljedal, I. B. Influence of the mutation 'diabetes' on insulin release and islet morphology in mice of different genetic backgrounds. *J. Cell. Biol.,* 1974, 62, 77-89.

[73] Baetens, D., Stefan, Y., Ravazzola, M., Malaisse-Lagae F., Coleman, D. L., Orci, L. Alteration of islet cell populations in spontaneously diabetic mice. *Diabetes*, 1978, 27, 1-7.

[74] Yokoi, N., Hoshino, M., Hidaka, S., Yoshida, E., Beppu, M., Hoshikawa, R., Sudo, K., Kawada, A., Takagi, S., Seino, S. A novel rat model of type 2 diabetes: the Zucker fatty diabetes mellitus ZFDM rat. *J. Diabetes Res.*, 2013, 2013, Article ID 103731, 9 pages. doi: /10.1155 103731/2013.

[75] Ashcroft, G. S., Horan, M. A., Ferguson, M. W. The effects of ageing on wound healing: immunolocalisation of growth factors and their receptors in a murine incisional model. *J. Anat.*, 1997, 190, 351-65.

[76] Hardman, M. J., Emmerson, E., Campbell, L., Ashcroft, G. S. Selective estrogen receptor modulators accelerate cutaneous wound healing in ovariectomized female mice. *Endocrinology*, 2008, 149, 551-7.

[77] Tatlidede, S., McCormack, M. C., Eberlin, K. R., Nguyen, J. T., Randolph, M. A., Austen, W. G., Jr. A novel murine island skin flap for ischemic preconditioning. *J. Surg. Res.,* 2009, 154, 112-7.

[78] Stadler, I., Zhang, R. Y., Oskoui, P., Whittaker, M. S., Lanzafame, R. J. Development of a simple, noninvasive, clinically relevant model of pressure ulcers in the mouse. *J. Invest. Surg.,* 2004, 17, 221-7.

[79] Kiran, K., Asad, M. Wound healing activity of *Sesamum indicum* L seed and oil in rats. *Indian J. Exp. Biol.*, 2008, 46, 777-82.

[80] Somboonwong, J., Kankaisre, M., Tantisira, B., Tantisira, M. H. Wound healing activities of different extracts of *Centella asiatica* in incision and burn wound models: an experimental animal study. *BMC Complement. Altern. Med.,* 2012, 12:103. doi:10.1186/1472-6882-12-103.

[81] Davidson, J. M. Animal models for wound repair. *Arch. Dermatol. Res.*, 1998, 290, S1-S11.

[82] Gottrup, F., Agren, M. S., Karlsmark, T. Models for use in wound healing research: a survey focusing on *in vitro* and *in vivo* adult soft tissue. *Wound Repair Regen.*, 2000, 8, 83-96.

[83] Nayak, S., Nalabothu, P., Sandiford, S., Bhogadi, V., Adogwa, A. Evaluation of wound healing activity of *Allamanda cathartica. L.* and *Laurus nobilis. L.* extracts on rats. *BMC Complement. Altern. Med.,* 2006, 6:12. doi:10.1186/1472-6882-6-12.

[84] Somboonwong, J., Thanamittramanee, S., Jariyapongskul, A., Patumraj, S. Therapeutic effects of *Aloe vera* on cutaneous microcirculation and wound healing in second degree burn model in rats. *J. Med. Assoc. Thai.*, 2000, 83, 417-25.

[85] Zawacki, B. E. Reversal of capillary stasis and prevention of necrosis in burns. *Ann. Surg.*, 1974, 180, 98-102.

[86] Knabl, J. S., Bayer, G. S., Bauer, W. A., Schwendenwein, I., Dado, P. F., Kucher, C., Horvat, R., Turkof, E., Schossmann, B., Meissl, G. Controlled partial skin thickness burns: an animal model for studies of burnwound progression. *Burns*, 1999, 25, 229-35.

[87] Tavares Pereira Ddos, S., Lima-Ribeiro, M. H., de Pontes-Filho, N. T., Carneiro-Leão, A. M., Correia, M. T. Development of animal model for studying deep second-degree thermal burns. *J. Biomed. Biotechnol.* 2012, 2012, 460841. doi:10.1155/2012/460841.

[88] Campelo, A. P., Campelo, M. W., Britto, G. A., Ayala, A. P., Guimarães, S. B., Vasconcelos, P. R. An optimized animal model for partial and total skin thickness burns studies. *Acta Cir. Bras.,* 2011, 26 (Suppl. 1), 38-42.

[89] Mitsunaga Junior, J. K., Gragnani, A., Ramos, M. L., Ferreira, L. M. Rat an experimental model for burns: a systematic review. *Acta Cir. Bras.*, 2012, 27, 417-23.

[90] Duansak, D., Somboonwong, J., Patumraj, S. Effects of *Aloe vera* on leukocyte adhesion and TNF-alpha and IL-6 levels in burn wounded rats. *Clin. Hemorheol. Microcirc.*, 2003, 29, 239-46.

[91] Kaushik, D., Kamboj, S., Kaushik, P., Sharma, S., Rana, A. C. Burn wound: Pathophysiology and its management by herbal plants. *Chron. Young Sci.,* 2013, 4, 86-93.

[92] Lehr, H. A., Leunig, M., Menger, M. D., Nolte, D., Messmer, K. Dorsal skinfold chamber technique for intravital microscopy in nude mice. *Am. J. Pathol.,* 1993, 143, 1055-62.

[93] Annan, K., Dickson, R. Evaluation of wound healing actions of *Hoslundia opposita* vahl, *Anthocleista nobilis* G. Don. and *Balanites aegyptiaca* L. *J. Sci. Technol.*, 2008, 28, 26-35.

[94] Barua, C. C., Talukda, A., Begum, S. A., Sarma, D. K., Pathak, D. C., Barua, A. G., Bora, R. S. Wound healing activity of methanolic extract of leaves of *Alternanthera brasilana* Kuntz using *in vivo* and in vitro model. *Indian J. Exp. Biol.,* 2009, 47, 1001-5.

[95] Bell, E., Sher, S., Hull, B., Merrill, C., Rosen, S., Chamson, A., Asselineau, D., Dubertret, L., Coulomb, B., Lapiere, C., Nusgens, B., Neveux, Y. The reconstitution of living skin. *J. Invest. Dermatol.*, 1983, 81, 2s-10s.

[96] Pistoor, F. H., Rambukkana, A., Kroezen, M., Lepoittevin, J. P., Bos, J. D., Kapsenberg, M. L., Das, P. K. Novel predictive assay for contact

allergens using human skin explant cultures. *Am. J. Pathol.*, 1996, 149, 337-43.

[97] Emanuelsson, P., Kratz, G. Characterization of a new in vitro burn wound model. *Burns,* 1997, 23, 32-6.

[98] Kratz, G. Modeling of wound healing processes in human skin using tissue culture. *Microsc. Res. Tech.*, 1998, 42, 345-50.

[99] Coolen, N. A., Vlig, M., van den Bogaerdt, A. J., Middelkoop, E., Ulrich, M. M. Development of an in vitro burn wound model. *Wound Repair Regen.*, 2008, 16, 559-67.

[100] Mathieu, D., Linke, J. C., Wattel, F. Non-healing wounds. In: Mathieu, D., editor. *Handbook on Hyperbaric Medicine*. Dordrecht: Springer; 2006; 401-27.

[101] Grindlay, D., Reynolds, T. The *Aloe vera* phenomenon: a review of the properties and modern uses of the leaf parenchyma gel. *J. Ethnopharmacol.*, 1986, 16, 117-51.

[102] Klein, A. D., Penneys, N. S. *Aloe vera. J. Am. Acad. Dermatol.*, 1988, 18, 714-20.

[103] Boudreau, M. D., Beland, F. A. An evaluation of the biological and toxicological properties of *Aloe Barbardensis* (Miller), *Aloe vera. J. Environ. Sci. Health C. Environ. Carcinog. Ecotoxicol. Rev.*, 2006, 24, 103-54.

[104] Gage, D. *Aloe vera*. Rochester, VT: Healing Arts Press; 1988.

[105] Rajeswari, R., Umadevi, M., Rahale, S. C., Pushpa, R., Selvavenkadesh, S., Kumar, K. P. S., Bhowmik, D. *Aloe vera*: the miracle plant its medicinal and traditional uses in India. *J. Pharmacogn. Phytochem.*, 2012, 1, 118-24.

[106] Primary Health Care, Ministry of Public Health of Thailand. *Herbs Used in Fundamental Public Health.* Bangkok: The War Veterans Organization of Thailand, 1998.

[107] Somboonwong, J., Duansak, N. The therapeutic efficacy and properties of topical *Aloe vera* in thermal burns. *J. Med. Assoc. Thai.*, 2004, 87, S.78-69

[108] Wilgus, T. A., Bergdall, V. K., Tober, K. L., Hill, K. J., Mitra, S., Flavahan, N. A., Oberyszyn, T M. The impact of cyclooxygenase-2 mediated inflammation on scarless fetal wound healing. *Am. J. Pathol.*, 2004, 165, 753-61.

[109] Fulton, J. E., Jr. The stimulation of postdermabrasion wound healing with stabilized *Aloe vera* gel-polyethylene oxide dressing. *J. Dermatol. Surg. Oncol.,* 1990, 16, 460-7.

[110] Lv, R. L., Wu, B. Y., Chen, X. D., Jiang, Q. The effects of aloe extract on nitric oxide and endothelin levels in deep-partial thickness burn wound tissue in rat. *Zhonghua Shao Shang Za Zhi.*, 2006, 22, 362-5.

[111] Somboonwong, J., Suwanmanee, S. *Aloe vera* and its microvascular affects on wound healing. In: Bunnag, S. C., Futrakul, P., Patumraj, S., editors. *Proceedings of 8th Asian Congress for Microcirculation: Microvascular Biology and Bioengineering towards Regenerative Medicine*. Bologna: Medimon; 2011; 81-84.

[112] Penneys, N. S. Inhibition of arachidonic acid oxidation *in vitro* by vehicle components. *Acta. Derm. Venereol.*, 1982, 62, 59-61.

[113] Heggers, J. P., Pelley, R. P., Robson, M. C. Beneficial effects of aloe in wound healing. *Phytother. Res.*, 1993, 7, S48-S52.

[114] Robson, M. C., Heggers, J. P., Hagstrom, W. J. Myth, magic, witchcraft or fact? *Aloe vera* revisited. *J. Burn Care Rehabil.*, 1982, 3, 157-63.

[115] Zawahry, M. E., Hegazy, M. R., Helal, M. Use of aloe in treating leg ulcers and dermatoses. *Int. J. Dermatol.,* 1973, 12, 68-73.

[116] Davis, R. H., DiDonato, J. J., Johnson, R. W., Stewart, C. B. *Aloe vera*, hydrocortisone, and sterol influence on wound tensile strength and anti-inflammation. *J. Am. Podiatr. Med. Assoc.*, 1994, 84, 614-21.

[117] Saito, H., Ishiguro, T., Imanishi, K., Suzuki, I. Pharmacological studies on a plant lectin aloctin A. II. Inhibitory effect of aloctin A on experimental models of inflammation in rats. *Jpn. J. Pharmacol.,* 1982, 32, 139-42.

[118] Ohuchi, K., Watanabe, M., Takahashi, E., Tsurufuji, S., Imanishi, K., Suzuki, I., Levine, L. Lectins modulate prostaglandin E2 production by rat peritoneal macrophages. *Agents Actions,* 1984, 15, 419-23.

[119] Davis, R. H., Kabbani, J. M., Maro, N. P. *Aloe vera* and inflammation. *Proc. Penn. Acad. Sci.*, 1986, 60, 67-70.

[120] Yagi, A., Kabash, A., Okamura, N., Haraguchi, H., Moustafa, S. M., Khalifa, T. I. Antioxidant, free radical scavenging and anti-inflammatory effects of aloesin derivatives in *Aloe vera*. *Planta. Med.*, 2002, 68, 957-60.

[121] Afzal, M., Ali, M., Hassan, R. A., Sweedan, N., Dhami, M. S. Identification of some prostanoids in *Aloe vera* extracts. *Planta. Med.*, 1991, 57, 38-40.

[122] Ro, J. Y., Lee, B. C., Kim, J. Y., Chung, Y. J., Chung, M. H., Lee, S. K., Jo, T. H., Kim, K. H., Park, Y. I. Inhibitory mechanism of aloe single component (alprogen) on mediator release in guinea pig lung mast cells

activated with specific antigen-antibody reactions. *J. Pharmacol. Exp. Ther.*, 2000, 292, 114-21.

[123] Fujita, K., Teradaira, R., Nagatsu, T. Bradykininase activity of aloe extract. *Biochem. Pharmacol.*, 1976, 25, 205.

[124] Fujita, K., Ito, S., Teradaira, R., Beppu, H. Properties of a carboxypeptidase from aloe. *Biochem. Pharmacol.*, 1979, 28, 1261-2.

[125] Rubel, B. L. Possible mechanism of the healing actions of aloe gel. *Cosmetics and Toiletries* 1983, 98, 109-14.

[126] Yagi, A., Harada, N., Yamada, H., Iwadare, S., Nishioka, I. Antibradykinin active material in *Aloe saponaria*. *J. Pharm. Sci.*, 1982, 71, 1172-4.

[127] Lehniger, A. *Biochemistry*. 2nd edition. New York: Worth Publishers Inc., 1977.

[128] Nakagomi, K., Oka, S., Tomizuka, N., Yamamoto, M., Masui, T., Nakazawa, H. Novel biological activities in *Aloe* components -- effects on mast cell degranulation and platelet aggregation. *Kenkyu Hokoku-Kogyo Gijutsuin Bisibutsu Kogyo*, 1985, 63, 3-9.

[129] Liu, X. S., Luo, Z. H., Yang, Z. C., Huang, W. H., Li, A. N. The significance of changes in serum tumour necrosis factor (TNF) activity in severely burned patients. *Burns,* 1994, 20, 40-4.

[130] Liu, X. S., Yang, Z. C., Luo, Z. H., Huang, W. H., Li, A. A preliminary exploration of the relationship between tumour necrosis factor) TNF (and monocytic *in vitro* production of interleukin-1) IL-1 (and internal organ dysfunction in severely burned patients. *Burns*, 1995, 21, 29-33.

[131] Arturson, G. Pathophysiology of the burn wound and pharmacological treatment. *Burns,* 1996, 22, 255-74.

[132] Deveci, M., Eski, M., Sengezer, M., Kisa, U. Effects of cerium nitrate bathing and prompt burn wound excision on IL-6 and TNF-alpha levels in burned rats. *Burns*, 2000, 26, 41-5.

[133] Vijayalakshmi, D., Dhandapani, R., Jayaveni, S., Jithendra, P. S., Rose, C., Mandal, A. B. In vitro anti-inflammatory activity of *Aloe vera* by down regulation of MMP-9 in peripheral blood mononuclear cells. *J. Ethnopharmacol.*, 2012, 141, 542-6.

[134] Grimble, R. F. Nutritional antioxidants and the modulation of inflammation: theory and practice. *New Horiz.*, 1994, 2, 175-85.

[135] Horton, J. W., White, D. J., Maass, D. L., Hybki, D. P., Haudek, S., Giroir, B. Antioxidant vitamin therapy alters burn trauma-mediated cardiac NF-kappaB activation and cardiomyocyte cytokine secretion. *J. Trauma*, 2001, 50, 397-406.

[136] Horton, J. W. Free radicals and lipid peroxidation mediated injury in burn trauma: the role of antioxidant therapy. *Toxicology*, 2003, 189, 75-88.

[137] Yagi, A., Kabash, A., Okamura, N., Haraguchi, H., Moustafa, S. M., Khalifa, T. I. Antioxidant, free radical scavenging and anti-inflammatory effects of aloesin derivatives in *Aloe vera. Planta. Med.*, 2002, 68, 957-60.

[138] Hu, Y., Xu, J., Hu, Q. Evaluation of antioxidant potential of *Aloe vera* (*Aloe barbadensis* Miller) extracts. *J. Agric. Food Chem.*, 2003, 51, 7788-91.

[139] Nejatzadeh-Barandozi, F. Antibacterial activities and antioxidant capacity of *Aloe vera. Org. Med. Chem. Lett.*, 2013, 3, 5. doi: /10.1186 .5-3-2858-2191

[140] Willenborg, D. O., Parish, C. R., Cowden, W. B. Phosphosugars are potent inhibitors of central nervous system inflammation. *FASEB J.*, 1989, 3, 1968-71.

[141] Coats, B. C., Ahola, R. J. *The Silent Healer -- A Modern Study of Aloe Vera.* Martinsville, IN: Fideli Publishing Inc., 2010.

[142] Parish, C. R., Willenborg, D. O., Cowden, W. B. Novel inhibitors of inflammation. *Today's Life Sci.,* 1990, 2, 20-7.

[143] Danhoff, I. E., McAnalley, B H. Stabilised *Aloe vera,* its effect on human skin cells. *Drug Cosmet. Ind.,* 1983, 133, 52-196.

[144] Davis, R. H., Maro, N. P. *Aloe vera* and gibberellin. Anti-inflammatory activity in diabetes. *J. Am. Podiatr. Med. Assoc.,* 1989, 79, 24-6.

[145] Hutter, J. A., Salman, M., Stavinoha, W. B., Satsangi, N., Williams, R. F., Streeper, R. T., Weintraub, S. T. Anti-inflammatory C-glucosyl chromone from *Aloe barbadensis. J. Nat. Prod.,* 1996, 59, 541-3.

[146] Brem, H., Jacobs, T., Vileikyte, L., Weinberger, S., Gibber, M., Gill, K., Tarnovskaya, A., Entero, H., Boulton, A. J. Wound-healing protocols for diabetic foot and pressure ulcers. *Surg. Technol. Int.*, 2003, 11, 85-92.

[147] Werner, S., Breeden, M., Hübner, G., Greenhalgh, D. G., Longaker, M. T. Induction of keratinocyte growth factor expression is reduced and delayed during wound healing in the genetically diabetic mouse. *J. Invest. Dermatol.,* 1994, 103, 469-73.

[148] Frank, S., Hübner, G., Breier, G., Longaker, M. T., Greenhalgh, D. G., Werner, S. Regulation of vascular endothelial growth factor expression in cultured keratinocytes. Implications for normal and impaired wound healing. *J. Biol. Chem.*, 1995, 270, 12607-13.

[149] Beer, H. D., Longaker, M. T., Werner, S. Reduced expression of PDGF and PDGF receptors during impaired wound healing. *J. Invest. Dermatol.,* 1997, 109, 132-8.

[150] Corral, C. J., Siddiqui, A., Wu, L., Farrell, C. L., Lyons, D., Mustoe, T. A. Vascular endothelial growth factor is more important than basic fibroblastic growth factor during ischemic wound healing. *Arch. Surg.*, 1999, 134, 200-5.

[151] Galiano, R. D., Tepper, O. M., Pelo, C. R., Bhatt, K. A., Callaghan, M., Bastidas, N., Bunting, S., Steinmetz, H. G., Gurtner, G. C. Topical vascular endothelial growth factor accelerates diabetic wound healing through increased angiogenesis and by mobilizing and recruiting bone marrow-derived cells. *Am. J. Pathol.*, 2004, 164, 1935-47.

[152] Li, W. W., Hutnik, M., Li, V. Angiogenesis-based medicine: principles and practice for disease prevention and intervention. In: Maragoudakis, M. E., Papadimitriou, E., editors. *Angiogenesis. Basic Science and Clinical Applications.* 1st edition. Kerala: Transworld Research Network; 2007; 337-417.

[153] Davis, R. H., Leitner, M. G., Russo, J. M., Byrne, M. E. Wound healing. Oral and topical activity of *Aloe vera. J. Am. Podiatr. Med. Assoc.*, 1989, 79, 559-62.

[154] Heggers, J. P., Pelley, R. P., Hill, D. P., Stabenau, C. J., Winters, W. D. Wound healing with aloe substances. *Academic/Industry Joint Conference*; 1992. p. 41.

[155] Tarameshloo, M., Norouzian, M., Zarein-Dolab, S., Dadpay, M., Mohsenifar, J., Gazor, R. *Aloe vera* gel and thyroid hormone cream may improve wound healing in Wistar rats. *Anat. Cell Biol.,* 2012, 45, 170-7.

[156] Atiba, A., Ueno, H., Uzuka, Y. The effects of *Aloe vera* oral administration on cutaneous wound healing in type 2 diabetic rats. *J. Vet. Med. Sci.*, 2011, 73, 583-9.

[157] Atiba, A., Nishimura, M., Kakinuma, S., Hiraoka, T., Goryo, M., Shimada, Y., Ueno, H., Uzuka, Y. *Aloe vera* oral administration accelerates acute radiation-delayed wound healing by stimulating transforming growth factor-ß and fibroblast growth factor production. *Am. J. Surg.*, 2011, 201, 809-18.

[158] Lee, M. J., Yoon, S. H., Lee, S. K., Chung, M. H., Park, Y. I., Sung, C. K., Choi, J. S., Kim, K. W. *In vivo* angiogenic activity of dichloromethane extracts of *Aloe vera* gel. *Arch. Pharm. Res.*, 1995, 18, 332-5.

[159] Lee, M. J., Lee, O. H., Yoon, S. H., Lee, S. K., Chung, M. H., Park, Y. I., Sung, C. K., Choi, J. S., Kim, K. W. *In vitro* angiogenic activity of *Aloe vera* gel on calf pulmonary artery endothelial (CPAE) cells. *Arch. Pharm. Res.*, 1998, 21, 260-5.

[160] Moon, E. J., Lee, Y. M., Lee, O. H., Lee, M. J., Lee, S. K., Chung, M. H., Park, Y. I., Sung, C. K., Choi, J. S., Kim, K. W. A novel angiogenic factor derived from *Aloe vera* gel: beta-sitosterol, a plant sterol. *Angiogenesis,* 1999, 3, 117-23.

[161] Choi, S., Kim, K. W., Choi, J. S., Han, S. T., Park, Y. I., Lee, S. K., Kim, J. S., Chung, M. H. Angiogenic activity of beta-sitosterol in the ischaemia/reperfusion-damaged brain of Mongolian gerbil. *Planta. Med.,* 2002, 68, 330-5.

[162] Jettanacheawchankit, S., Sasithanasate, S., Sangvanich, P., Banlunara, W., Thunyakitpisal, P. Acemannan stimulates gingival fibroblast proliferation; expressions of keratinocyte growth factor-1, vascular endothelial growth factor, and type I collagen; and wound healing. *J. Pharmacol. Sci.,* 2009, 109, 525-31.

[163] Laplante, A. F., Germain, L., Auger, F. A., Moulin, V. Mechanisms of wound reepithelialization: hints from a tissue-engineered reconstructed skin to long-standing questions. *FASEB J.,* 2001, 15, 2377-89.

[164] Abdul-Samad, M. A., Kadhum, M. A., Hamza, B. S., Hamed, M. M. The effect of *Aloe vera* acetone extract on wound contraction and re-epithelialization on full-thickness excisional wound in female rabbits. *AL-Qadisiya J. Vet. Med. Sci.,* 2008, 7, 44-49.

[165] Bunyapraphatsara, N., Jirakulchaiwong, S., Thirawarapan, S., Manonukul, J. The efficacy of *Aloe vera* cream in the treatment of first, second and third degree burns in mice. *Phytomedicine*, 1996, 2, 247-51.

[166] Hosseinimehr, S. J., Khorasani, G., Azadbakht, M., Zamani, P., Ghasemi, M., Ahmadi, A. Effect of aloe cream versus silver sulfadiazine for healing burn wounds in rats. *Acta Dermatovenerol. Croat.*, 2010, 18, 2-7.

[167] Shahzad, M. N., Ahmed, N. Effectiveness of *Aloe vera* gel compared with 1% silver sulphadiazine cream as burn wound dressing in second degree burns. *J. Pak. Med. Assoc.*, 2013, 63, 225-30.

[168] Choi, S. W., Son, B. W., Son, Y. S., Park, Y. I., Lee, S. K., Chung, M. H. The wound-healing effect of a glycoprotein fraction isolated from aloe vera. *Br. J. Dermatol.*, 2001, 145, 535-45.

[169] Inpanya, P., Faikrua, A., Ounaroon, A., Sittichokechaiwut, A., Viyoch, J. Effects of the blended fibroin/aloe gel film on wound healing in

streptozotocin-induced diabetic rats. *Biomed. Mater.*, 2012, 7(3):035008. doi: 10.1088/1748-6041/7/3/035008.

[170] Chithra, P., Sajithlal, G. B., Chandrakasan, G. Influence of *Aloe vera* on the glycosaminoglycans in the matrix of healing dermal wounds in rats. *J. Ethnopharmacol*, 1998a, 59, 179-86.

[171] Chithra, P., Sajithlal, G. B., Chandrakasan, G. Influence of *Aloe vera* on collagen characteristics in healing dermal wounds in rats. *Mol. Cell Biochem.*, 1998, 181, 71-6.

[172] Chithra, P., Sajithlal, G. B., Chandrakasan, G. Influence of *Aloe vera* on collagen turnover in healing of dermal wounds in rats. *Indian J. Exp. Biol.*, 1998, 36, 896-901.

[173] Chithra, P., Sajithlal, B., Chandrakasan, G. Influence of *Aloe vera* on the healing of dermal wounds in diabetic rats. *J. Ethnopharmacol.*, 1998b, 59, 195-201.

[174] Oryan, A., Mohammadalipour, A., Moshiri, A., Tabandeh, M. R. Topical application of *Aloe vera* accelerated wound healing, modeling, and remodeling: an experimental study with significant clinical value. *Ann. Plast. Surg.*, 2014, [Epub. ahead of print].

[175] Abdullah, K. M., Abdullah, A., Johnson, M. L., Bilski, J. J., Petry, K., Redmer, D. A., Reynolds, L. P., Grazul-Bilska, A. T. Effects of *Aloe vera* on gap junctional intercellular communication and proliferation of human diabetic and nondiabetic skin fibroblasts. *J. Altern. Complement. Med.,* 2003, 9, 711-8.

[176] Yao, H., Chen, Y., Huang, L., Chen, W., Lin, X. Promotion proliferation effect of a polysaccharide from *Aloe barbadensis* Miller on human fibroblasts *in vitro. Int. J. Biol. Macromol.*, 2009, 45, 152-6.

[177] Liu, L. Y., Chen, X. D., Wu, B. Y., Jiang, Q. Influence of Aloe polysaccharide on proliferation and hyaluronic acid and hydroxyproline secretion of human fibroblasts *in vitro. Zhong Xi Yi Jie He Xue Bao*, 2010, 8, 256-62.

[178] Morgan, D. O., Edman, J. C., Standring, D. N., Fried, V. A., Smith, M. C., Roth, R. A., Rutter, W. J. Insulin-like growth factor II receptor as a multifunctional binding protein. *Nature*, 1987, 329, 301-7.

[179] Braulke, T., Causin, C., Waheed, A., Junghans, U., Hasilik, A., Maly, P., Humbel, R. E., von Figura, K. Mannose 6-phosphate/insulin-like growth factor II receptor: distinct binding sites for mannose 6-phosphate and insulin-like growth factor II. *Biochem. Biophys. Res. Commun.*, 1988, 150, 1287-93.

[180] Winters, W., Benavides, R., Clouse, W. J. Effects of aloe extracts on human normal and tumor cells *in vitro*. *Econ. Bot.*, 1981, 35, 89-95.
[181] Yagi, A., Egusa, T., Arase, M., Tanabe, M., Tsuji, H. Isolation and characterization of the glycoprotein fraction with a proliferation-promoting activity on human and hamster cells *in vitro* from *Aloe vera* gel. *Planta Med.,* 1997, 63, 18-21.
[182] Topman, G., Lin, F. H., Gefen, A. The natural medications for wound healing – Curcumin, *Aloe-Vera* and Ginger – do not induce a significant effect on the migration kinematics of cultured fibroblast. *J. Biomech.*, 2013, 46, 170-4.
[183] Engel, E. D., Erlick, N. E., Davis, R. H. Diabetes mellitus: impaired wound healing from zinc deficiency. *J. Am. Podiatry Assoc.*, 1981, 71, 536-44.
[184] Barrantes, E., Guinea, M. Inhibition of collagenase and metalloproteinases by aloins and aloe gel. *Life Sci.*, 2003, 72, 843-50.
[185] Tabandeh, M. R., Oryan, A., Mohammadalipour, A. Polysaccharides of *Aloe vera* induce MMP-3 and TIMP-2 gene expression during the skin wound repair of rat. *Int. J. Biol. Macromol.*, 2014, 65, 424-30.
[186] Ferro, V. A., Bradbury, F., Cameron, P., Shakir, E., Rahman, S. R., Stimson, W. H. *In vitro* susceptibilities of *Shigella flexneri* and *Streptococcus pyogenes* to inner gel of *Aloe barbadensis* Miller. *Antimicrob. Agents Chemother.*, 2003, 47, 1137-9.
[187] Agarry, O. O., Olaleye, M. T., Bello-Michael, C. O. Comparative antimicrobial activities of *Aloe vera* gel and leaf. *Afr. J. Biotechnol.*, 2005, 4, 1413-4.
[188] Pawar, V. C., Bagatharia, S. B., Thaker, V. S., Antibacterial activity of *Aloe vera* leaf gel extracts against *Staphylococcus aureus*. *Indian J. Microbiol.*, 2005, 45, 227-9.
[189] Lawrence, R., Tripathi, P., Jeyakumar, E. Isolation, purification and evaluation of antibacterial agents from *Aloe vera*. *Braz. J. Microbiol.*, 2009, 40, 906-15.
[190] Arunkumar, S., Muthuselvam, M. Analysis of phytochemical constituents and antimicrobial activities of *Aloe vera* L. against clinical pathogens. *World J. Agric. Sci.,* 2009, 5, 572-6.
[191] Thiruppathi, S., Ramasubramanian, V., Sivakumar, T., Thirumalai Arasu, V. Antimicrobial activity of *Aloe vera* (L.) Burm. f. against pathogenic microorganisms. *J. Biosci. Res.*, 2010, 1, 251-8.

[192] Athiban, P. P., Borthakur, B. J., Ganesan, S., Swathika, B. Evaluation of antimicrobial efficacy of *Aloe vera* and its effectiveness in decontaminating gutta percha cones. *J. Conserv. Dent.*, 2012, 15, 246-8.

[193] Rodiguez-Bigas, M., Cruz, N. I., Suárez, A. Comparative evaluation of *Aloe vera* in the management of burn wounds in guinea pigs. *Plast. Reconstr. Surg.*, 1988, 81, 386-9.

[194] Kivett, W. F. *Aloe vera* for burns. *Plast. Reconstr. Surg.*, 1989, 83, 195.

[195] Cera, L. M., Heggers, J. P., Robson, M. C., Hagstrom, W. J. The therapeutic efficacy of *Aloe vera* cream (Dermaide Aloe®) in thermal injuries: two case reports. *J. Am. Anim. Hosp. Assoc.*, 1980, 16, 768-72.

[196] Heck, E., Head, M., Novak, D., Helm, P., Baxter, C. *Aloe vera* (gel) cream as a topical treatment for outpatient burns. *Burns*, 1981, 7, 291-4.

[197] Heggers, J. P., Kucukcelebi, A., Listengarten, D., Stabenau, J., Ko, F., Broemeling, L. D., Robson, M. C., Winters, W. D. Beneficial effect of Aloe on wound healing in an excisional wound model. *J. Altern. Complement. Med.*, 1996, 2, 271-7.

[198] Muller, M. J., Hollyoak, M. A., Moaveni, Z., Brown, T. L., Herndon, D. N., Heggers, J. P. Retardation of wound healing by silver sulfadiazine is reversed by *Aloe vera* and nystatin. *Burns*, 2003, 29, 834-6.

[199] Cuttle, L., Kempf, M., Kravchuk, O., George, N., Liu, P. Y., Chang, H. E., Mill, J., Wang, X. Q., Kimble, R. M. The efficacy of *Aloe vera*, tea tree oil and saliva as first aid treatment for partial thickness burn injuries. *Burns*, 2008, 34, 1176-82.

[200] Azghani, A. O., Williams, I., Holiday, D. B., Johnson, A. R. A beta-linked mannan inhibits adherence of *Pseudomonas aeruginosa* to human lung epithelial cells. *Glycobiology,* 1995, 5, 39-44.

[201] Kahlon, J. B., Kemp, M. C., Yawei, N., Carpenter, R. H., Shannon, W. M., McAnalley, B. H. *In vitro* evaluation of the synergistic antiviral effects of acemannan in combination with azidothymidine and acyclovir. *Mol. Biother.*, 1991, 3, 214-23.

[202] Kemp, M. C., Kahlon, J. B., Chinnah, A. D., Carpenter, R. H., McAnalley, B. H., McDaniel, H. R., Shannon, W. M. *In vitro* evaluation of the antiviral effects of acemannan on the replication and pathogenesis of HIV-1 and other enveloped viruses: modification of the processing of glycoprotein precursors. *Antiviral Res.*, 1990, 13, 83.

[203] Pugh, N., Ross, S. A., ElSohly, M. A., Pasco, D. S. Characterization of Aloeride, a new high-molecular-weight polysaccharide from *Aloe vera* with potent immunostimulatory activity. *J. Agric. Food Chem.*, 2001, 49: 1030-4.

[204] Heggers, J. P., Kucukcelebi, A., Stabenau, C. J., Ko, F., Broemeling, L. D., Robson, M. C., Winters, W. D. Wound healing effects of Aloe gel and other topical antibacterial agents on rat skin. *Phytother. Res.*, 1995, 9, 455-7.

[205] Erazo, S., Lemus, I., Garcia, R. Evaluation of the humectant properties of *Aloe perryi* Baker. *Plantes. Med. Phytother.*, 1985, 19, 240-7.

[206] Davis, R. H., Parker, W. L., Samson, R. T., Murdoch, D. P. The isolation of an active inhibitory system from an extract of *Aloe Vera*. *J. Am. Podiatr. Med. Assoc.,* 1991, 81, 258-61.

[207] Davis, R. H., Parker, W. L., Samson, R. T., Murdoch, D. P. Isolation of a stimulatory system in an Aloe extract. *J. Am. Podiatr. Med. Assoc.,* 1991, 81, 473-8.

[208] Tizard, I. R., Carpenter, R. H., McAnalley, B. H., Kemp, M. C. The biological activities of mannans and related complex carbohydrates. *Mol. Biother.*, 1989, 1, 290-6.

[209] Maxwell, B., Chinnah, H., Tizard, I. Activated macrophages accelerate wound healing in aged rats. *Wound Repair Regen.*, 1996, 4, 165.

[210] Farahnejad, Z., Ghazanfari, T., Yaraee, R. Immunomodulatory effects of *Aloe vera* and its fractions on response of macrophages against *Candida albicans*. *Immunopharmacol. Immunotoxicol.*, 2011, 33, 676-81.

[211] Madan, J., Sharma, A. K., Inamdar, N., Rao, H. S., Singh, R . Immunomodulatory properties of *Aloe vera* gel in mice. *Int. J. Green. Pharm.*, 2008, 2, 152-4.

[212] Im, S. A., Lee, Y. R., Lee, Y. H., Lee, M. K., Park, Y. I., Lee, S., Kim, K., Lee, C. K. *In vivo* evidence of the immunomodulatory activity of orally administered *Aloe vera* gel. *Arch. Pharm. Res.*, 2010, 33, 451-6.

[213] Karaca, K., Sharma, J. M., Nordgren, R. Nitric oxide production by chicken macrophages activated by Acemannan, a complex carbohydrate extracted from *Aloe vera*. *Int. J. Immunopharmacol.*, 1995, 17, 183-8.

[214] Zhang, L., Tizard, I. R. Activation of a mouse macrophage cell line by acemannan: the major carbohydrate fraction from *Aloe vera* gel. *Immunopharmacology*, 1996, 35, 119-28.

[215] Ramamoorthy, L., Kemp, M. C., Tizard, I R. Acemannan, a beta-(1,4)-acetylated mannan, induces nitric oxide production in macrophage cell line RAW 264.7. *Mol. Pharmacol.*, 1996, 50, 878-84.

[216] Takata, I., Chida, K., Gordon, M. R., Myrvik, Q. N., Ricardo, M. J. Jr; Kucera, L. S. L-fucose, D-mannose, L-galactose, and their BSA conjugates stimulate macrophage migration. *J. Leukoc. Biol.,* 1987, 41, 248-56.

[217] Im, S. A., Oh, S. T., Song, S., Kim, M. R., Kim, D. S., Woo, S. S., Jo, T. H., Park, Y. I., Lee, C. K. Identification of optimal molecular size of modified Aloe polysaccharides with maximum immunomodulatory activity. *Int. Immunopharmacol.*, 2005, 5, 271-9.

[218] Sarkar, D., Dutta, A., Das, M., Sarkar, K., Mandal, C., Chatterjee, M. Effect of *Aloe vera* on nitric oxide production by macrophages during inflammation. *Indian J. Pharmacol.*, 2005, 37, 371-5.

[219] Budai, M. M., Varga, A., Milesz, S., Tőzsér, J., Benkő, S. *Aloe vera* downregulates LPS-induced inflammatory cytokine production and expression of NLRP3 inflammasome in human macrophages. *Mol. Immunol.,* 2013, 56, 471-9.

[220] Vogler, B. K., Ernst, E. *Aloe vera*: a systematic review of its clinical effectiveness. *Br. J. Gen. Pract.*, 1999, 49, 823-8.

[221] Schmidt, J. M., Greenspoon, J. S. *Aloe vera* dermal wound gel is associated with a delay in woung healing. *Obstet. Gynecol.*, 1991, 78, 115-7.

[222] Maenthaisong, R., Chaiyakunapruk, N., Niruntraporn, S., Kongkaew, C. The efficacy of *Aloe vera* used for burn wound healing: A systematic review. *Burns*, 2007, 33, 713-8.

[223] Thamlikitkul, V., Bunyapraphatsara, N., Riewpailboon, W., Theerapong, S., Chantrakul, C., Thanaveerasuwan, T., Nimitnon, S., Wongkonkatape, S., Riewpaiboon, A., Tenambergen, E. D. Clinical trial of *Aloe vera* Linn. for treatment of minor burns. *Siriraj Hosp. Gaz.*, 1991, 43, 313-6.

[224] Visuthikosol, V., Chowcheun, C., Sukwanarat, Y., Sriurairatana, S., Boonpugnavig, V. Effect of *Aloe vera* gel to healing of burn wound: a clinical and histologic study. *J. Med. Assoc. Thai.*, 1995, 78, 403-9.

[225] Akhtar, M. A., Hatwar, S. K. Efficacy of *Aloe vera* extract cream in management of burn wound. *J. Clin. Epidemiol.*, 1996, 49 (Suppl. 1), 24.

[226] Sun, J. H., Chen, X. G., Jin, R. T., Li, T. N., Bian, Y. X. People's Liberation Army medicine information. *Med. J. Chin. Army*, 1994, 8, 191-2.

[227] Dat, A. D., Poon, F., Pham, K. B., Doust, J. *Aloe vera* for treating acute and chronic wounds. *Cochrane Database Syst. Rev.,* 2012, 2:CD008762. doi: 10.1002/14651858.CD008762.pub2.

[228] Khorasani, G., Hosseinimehr, S. J., Azadbakht, M., Zamani, A., Mahdavi, M. R. Aloe versus silver sulfadiazine creams for second-degree burns: a randomized controlled study. *Surg. Today,* 2009, 39, 587-91.

[229] Eshghi, F., Hosseinimehr, S. J., Rahmani, N., Khademloo, M., Norozi, M. S., Hojati, O. Effects of *Aloe vera* cream on posthemorrhoidectomy pain and wound healing :results of a randomized, blind, placebo-control study. *J. Altern. Complement. Med.*, 2010, 16, 647-50.

[230] Phillips, T., Ongenae, K., Kanj, L., Slater-Freedberg, J. A randomised study of an *Aloe vera* derivative gel dressing versus conventional treatment after shave biopsy excisions. *Wounds*, 1995, 7, 200-2.

[231] Thomas, D. R., Goode, P. S., LaMaster, K., Tennyson, T. Acemannan hydrogel dressing versus saline dressing for pressure ulcers: a randomized, controlled trial. *Adv. Wound Care*, 1998, 11, 273-6.

[232] Shahzad, M. N., Ahmed, N. Effectiveness of *Aloe Vera* gel compared with 1% silver sulphadiazine cream as burn wound dressing in second degree burns. *J. Pak. Med. Assoc.*, 2013, 63, 225-30.

[233] World Health Organization. *WHO Monographs on Selected Medicinal Plants.* Volume 1. Geneva: World Health Organization, 1999.

[234] Zheng, C. J., Qin, L. P. Chemical components of *Centella asiatica* and their bioactivities. *J. Chin. Integr. Med.*, 2007, 5, 348-51.

[235] Kosalwatna, S., Shaipanich, C., Bhanganada, K., The effect of one percent *Centella asiatica* cream on chronic ulcers. *Siriraj Hosp. Gaz.*, 1988, 40, 455-61.

[236] Paocharoen, V. The efficacy and side effects of oral *Centella asiatica* extract for wound healing promotion in diabetic wound patients. *J. Med. Assoc. Thai.,* 2010, 93, S166-70.

[237] Chen, Y. J., Dai, Y. S., Chen, B. F., Chang, A., Chen, H. C., Lin, Y. C., Chang, K. H., Lai, Y. L., Chung, C. H., Lai, Y. J. The effect of tetrandrine and extracts of *Centella asiatica* on acute radiation dermatitis in rats. *Biol. Pharm. Bull.* 1999, 22, 703-6.

[238] Maquart, F. X., Chastang, F., Simeon, A., Birembaut, P., Gillery, P., Wegrowski, Y. Triterpenes from *Centella asiatica* stimulate extracellular matrix accumulation in rat experimental wounds. *Eur. J. Dermatol.,* 1999, 9, 289-96.

[239] Shetty, B. S., Udupa, S. L., Udupa, A. L., Somayaji, S. N. Effect of *Centella asiatica* L (Umbelliferae) on normal and dexamethasone-suppressed wound healing in Wistar Albino rats. *Int. J. Low. Extrem. Wounds,* 2006, 5, 137-43.

[240] Liu, M., Dai, Y., Li, Y., Luo, Y., Huang, F., Gong, Z., Meng, Q. Madecassoside isolated from *Centella asiatica* herbs facilitates burn wound healing in mice. *Planta Med.,* 2008, 74, 809-15.

[241] Chong, N. J., Aziz, Z. A systematic review of the efficacy of *Centella asiatica* for improvement of the signs and symptoms of chronic venous insufficiency. *Evid-Based Compl. Alt.*, 2013, 2013, 627182. doi: 10. 1155/2013/627182.

[242] Somchit, M. N., Sulaiman, M. R., Zuraini, A., Samsuddin, L., Somchit, N., Israf, D. A., Moin, S. Antinociceptive and antiinflammatory effects of *Centella asiatica. Indian J. Pharmacol.*, 2004, 36, 377-80.

[243] Yun, K. J., Kim, J. Y., Kim, J. B., Lee, K. W., Jeong, S. Y., Park, H. J., Jung, H. J., Cho, Y. W., Yun, K., Lee, K. T. Inhibition of LPS-induced NO and PGE2 production by asiatic acid via NF-kappa B inactivation in RAW 264.7 macrophages: possible involvement of the IKK and MAPK pathways. *Int. Immunopharmacol.*, 2008, 8: 431-41.

[244] Won, J. H., Shin, J. S., Park, H. J., Jung, H. J., Koh, D. J., Jo, B. G., Lee, J. Y., Yun, K., Lee, K. T. Anti-inflammatory effects of madecassic acid via the suppression of NF-kappa B pathway in LPS-induced RAW 264.7 macrophage cells. *Planta Med.*, 2010, 76, 251-7.

[245] Nurlaily, A., Noor Baitee, A. R., Musalmah, M. Comparative antioxidant and anti-inflammatory activity of different extracts of *Centella asiatica* (L.) Urban and its active compounds, asiaticoside and madecassoside. *Med. and Health*, 2012, 7, 62-72.

[246] George, M., Joseph, L., Ramaswamy. Anti-allergic, anti-pruritic, and anti-inflammatory activities of *Centella asiatica* extracts. *Afr. J. Tradit. Complement. Altern. Med.*, 2009, 6: 554-9.

[247] Saha, S., Guria, T., Singha, T., Maity, T. K. Evaluation of analgesic and anti-Inflammatory activity of chloroform and methanol extracts of *Centella asiatica* Linn. *ISRN Pharmacol.*, 2013, 2013, 789613. doi: 10. 1155/2013/789613.

[248] Coldren, C. D., Hashim, P., Ali, J. M., Oh, S. K., Sinskey, A. J., Rha, C. Gene expression changes in the human fibroblast induced by *Centella asiatica* triterpenoids. *Planta Med.,* 2003, 69, 725-32.

[249] Anand, T., Naika, M., Kumar, P. G, Khanum, F. Antioxidant and DNA damage preventive properties of *Centella asiatica* (L) Urb. *Phcog. J.*, 2010, 2, 53-8.

[250] Rahman, M., Hossain, S., Rahaman, A., Fatima, N., Nahar, T., Uddin, B, Basunia, M. A. Antioxidant activity of *Centella asiatica* (Linn.) Urban: impact of extraction solvent polarity. *J. Pharmacogn. Phytochem.*, 2013, 1, 27-32.

[251] Chippada, S. C., Volluri, S. S., Bammidi, S. R, Vangalapati, M. *In vitro* anti-inflammatory activity of methanolic extract of *Centella asiatica* by HRBC membrane stabilization. *Rasayan J. Chem.*, 2011, 4, 457-60.

[252] Shukla, A., Rasik, A. M., Jain, G. K., Shankar, R., Kulshrestha, D. K., Dhawan, B. N. *In vitro* and *in vivo* wound healing activity of asiaticoside isolated from *Centella asiatica. J. Ethnopharmacol.*, 1999, 65, 1-11.

[253] Kimura, Y., Sumiyoshi, M., Samukawa, K., Satake, N., Sakanaka, M. Facilitating action of asiaticoside at low doses on burn wound repair and its mechanism. *Eur. J. Pharmacol.*, 2008, 584, 415-23.

[254] Suguna, L., Sivakumar, P., Chandrakasan, G. Effects of *Centella asiatica* extract on dermal wound healing in rats. *Indian J. Exp. Biol.*, 1996, 34, 1208-11.

[255] Sunikumar, Parameshwaraiah, S., Shivakumar, H. G. Evaluation of topical formulations of aqueous extract of *Centella asiatica* on open wounds in rats. *Indian J. Exp. Biol.*, 1998, 36, 569-72.

[256] Tenni, R., Zanaboni, G., De Agostini, M. P., Rossi, A., Bendotti, C., Cetta, G. Effect of the triterpenoid fraction of *Centella asiatica* on macromolecules of the connective matrix in human skin fibroblast cultures. *Ital. J. Biochem.*, 1988, 37, 69-77.

[257] Hashim, P. The effect of *Centella asiatica*, vitamins, glycolic acid and their mixtures preparations in stimulating collagen and fibronectin synthesis in cultured human skin fibroblast. *Pak. J. Pharm. Sci.*, 2014, 27, 233-7.

[258] Lu, L., Ying, K., Wei, S., Fang, Y., Liu, Y., Lin, H., Ma, L., Mao, Y. Asiaticoside induction for cell-cycle progression, proliferation and collagen synthesis in human dermal fibroblasts. *Int. J. Dermatol.,* 2004, 43, 801-7.

[259] Bonté, F., Dumas, M., Chaudagne, C., Meybeck, A. Asiaticoside and madecassoside activity on human fibroblast type I and III collagen secretion. *Ann. Pharm. Fr.*, 1995, 53; 38-42.

[260] Wu, F., Bian, D., Xia, Y., Gong, Z., Tan, Q., Chen, J., Dai, Y. Identification of major active ingredients responsible for burn wound healing of *Centella asiatica* herbs. *Evid. Based Complement. Alternat. Med.*, 2012, 2012, .848093doi: 848093/2012/10.1155.

[261] Lee, J. H., Kim, H. L., Lee, M. H., You, K. E., Kwon, B. J., Seo, H. J., Park, J. C. Asiaticoside enhances normal human skin cell migration, attachment and growth *in vitro* wound healing model. *Phytomedicine*, 2012, 19, 1223-7.

[262] Wysocki, A. B., Kusakabe, A. O., Chang, S., Tuan, T. L. Temporal expression pf urokinase plasminogen activator, plasminogen activator inhibitor and gelatinase-B in chronic wound fluid switches from a chronic to acute wound profile with progression to healing. *Wound Repair Regen.*, 1999, 7, 154-65.

[263] Lee, E., Vaughan, D. E., Parikh, S. H., Grodzinsky, A. J., Libby, P., Lark, M. W., Lee, R. T. Regulation of matrix metalloproteinases and plasminogen activator inhibitor-1 synthesis by plasminogen in cultured human vascular smooth muscle cells. *Cir. Res.*, 1996, 78, 44-9.

[264] Varga, J., Rosenbloom, J., Jimenez, S. A. Transforming growth factor beta (TGF beta) causes a persistent increase in steady-state amounts of type I and type III collagen and fibronectin mRNAs in normal human dermal fibroblasts. *Biochem. J.*, 1987, 247, 597-604.

[265] Lee, J., Jung, E., Kim, Y., Park, J., Park, J., Hong, S., Kim, J., Hyun, C., Kim, Y. S., Park, D. Asiaticoside induces human collagen I synthesis through TGFbeta receptor I kinase (TbetaRI kinase)-independent Smad signaling. *Planta Med.*, 2006, 72, 324-8.

[266] Shukla, A., Rasik, A. M., Dhawan, B. N. Asiaticoside-induced elevation of antioxidant levels in healing wounds. *Phytother. Res.*, 1999, 13, 50-4.

[267] Nema, N K., Maity, N., Sarkar, B. K., Mukherjee, P. K. Matrix metalloproteinase, hyaluronidase and elastase inhibitory potential of standardized extract of *Centella asiatica*. *Pharm. Biol.*, 2013, 51, 1182-7.

[268] May, A. The effect of asiaticoside on pig skin in organ culture. *Eur. J. Pharmacol.*, 1968, 4, 331-9.

[269] Lee, T. Y., Chin, G. S., Kim, W. J., Chau, D., Gittes, G. K., Longaker, M. T. Expression of transforming growth factor beta 1, 2, and 3 proteins in keloids. *Ann. Plast. Surg.*, 1999, 43, 179-84.

[270] Baker, R., Urso-Baiarda, F., Linge, C., Grobbelaar, A. Cutaneous scarring: a clinical review. *Dermatol. Res. Pract.*, 2009, 2009, 625376. doi:10.1155/2009/625376.

[271] Widgerow, A. D., Chait, L. A., Stals, P. J. New innovations in scar management. *Aesthetic Plast. Surg.*, 2000, 24, 227-34.

[272] Zhang, T., Rong, X. Z., Yang, R. H., Li, T. Z., Xu, Y. B. Effect of asiaticoside on the expression of transforming growth factor-beta mRNA and matrix metalloproteinases in hypertrophic scars. *J. Southern Medical University*, 2006, 26, 67-70.

[273] Xie, J., Qi, S., Li, T., Huang, B., Tang, J., Xu, Y., Liu, X., Shu, B., Liang, H., Huang, Y. Effect of asiaticoside on hypertrophic scar in the rabbit ear model. *J. Cutan. Pathol.*, 2009, 36, 234-9.

[274] Tang, B., Zhu, B., Liang, Y., Bi, L., Hu, Z., Chen, B., Zhang, K., Zhu, J. Asiaticoside suppresses collagen expression and TGF-β/Smad signaling through inducing Smad7 and inhibiting TGF-βRI and TGF-βRII in keloid fibroblasts. *Arch. Dermatol. Res.*, 2011, 303, 563-72.

[275] Bian, D., Zhang, J., Wu, X., Dou, Y., Yang, Y., Tan, Q., Xia, Y., Gong, Z., Dai, Y. Asiatic acid isolated from *Centella asiatica* inhibits TGF-βI-induced collagen expression in human keloid fibroblasts via PPAR-γ activation. *Int. J. Biol. Sci.,* 2013, 9, 1032-42. doi:10.7150/ijbs.7273.

[276] El-Hefnawi, H. Treatment of keloid with asiaticoside. *Dermatologica,* 1962, 125, 387-92.

[277] Morisset, R., Côté, N. G., Panisset, J. C., Jemni, L., Camirand, P., Brodeur, A. Evaluation of the healing activity of hydrocotyle tincture in the treatment of wounds. *Phytother. Res.,* 1987, 1, 117-21.

[278] Song, J., Xu, H., Lu, Q., Xu, Z., Bian, D., Xia, Y., Wei, Z., Gong, Z., Dai, Y. Madecassoside suppresses migration of fibroblasts from keloids: involvement of p38 kinase and PI3K signaling pathways. *Burns,* 2012, 38: 677-84.

[279] European Scientific Cooperative on Phytotherapy (ESCOP). *ESCOP Monographs: The Scientific Foundation for Herbal Medicinal Products.* New York, NY: Thieme, 2003.

[280] Dash, B. K., Faruquee, H. M., Biswas, S. K., Alam, M. K., Sisir, S. M., Prodhan, U. K. Antibacterial and antifungal activities of several extracts of *Centella asiatica* L. against some human pathogenic microbes. *Life Sci. Med. Res.*, 2011, 35, 1-5.

[281] Zaidan, M. R., Noor Rain, A., Badrul, A. R., Adlin, A., Norazah, A., Zakiah, I. *In vitro* screening of five local medicinal plants for antibacterial activity using disc diffusion method. *Trop. Biomed.*, 2005, 22, 165-70.

[282] Fugh-Berman, A. *The 5-minute herb and dietary supplement consult.* Philadelphia, PA: Lippincott Williams and Wilkins, 2003.

[283] Sidhu, G. S., Singh, A. K., Thaloor, D., Banaudha, K. K., Patnaik, G. K., Srimal, R. C., Maheshwari, R. K. Enhancement of wound healing by curcumin in animals. *Wound Repair Regen.*, 1998, 6, 167-77.

[284] Kulac, M., Aktas, C., Tulubas, F., Uygur, R., Kanter, M., Erboga, M., Ceber, M., Topcu, B., Ozen, O. A. The effects of topical treatment with

curcumin on burn wound healing in rats. *J. Mol. Histol.*, 2013, 44, 83-90.

[285] Singer, A. J., McClain, S. A., Romanov, A., Rooney, J., Zimmerman, T. Curcumin reduces burn progression in rats. *Acad. Emerg. Med.*, 2007, 14, 1125-9.

[286] Singer, A. J., Taira, B. R., Lin, F., Lim, T., Anderson, R., McClain, S. A., Clark, R. A. Curcumin reduces injury progression in a rat comb burn model. *J. Burn Care Res.*, 2011, 32, 135-42.

[287] Sidhu, G. S., Mani, H., Gaddipati, J. P., Singh, A. K., Seth, P., Banaudha, K. K., Patnaik, G. K., Maheshwari, R. K. Curcumin enhances wound healing in streptozotocin induced diabetic rats and genetically diabetic mice. *Wound Repair Regen.*, 1999, 7, 362-74.

[288] Jagetia, G. C., Rajanikant, G. K. Effect of curcumin on radiation-impaired healing of excisional wounds in mice. *J. Wound Care*, 2004, 13, 107-9.

[289] Jagetia, G. C., Rajanikant, G. K. Role of curcumin, a naturally occurring phenolic compound of turmeric in accelerating the repair of excision wound, in mice whole-body exposed to various doses of gamma-radiation. *J. Surg. Res.*, 2004, 120, 127-38.

[290] Jagetia, G. C., Rajanikant, G. K. Curcumin treatment enhances the repair and regeneration of wounds in mice exposed to hemibody gamma-irradiation. *Plast. Reconstr. Surg.*, 2005, 115, 515-28.

[291] Jagetia, G. C., Rajanikant, G. K. Acceleration of wound repair by curcumin in the excision wound of mice exposed to different doses of fractionated γ radiation. *Int. Wound J.*, 2012, 9, 76-92.

[292] López-Jornet, P., Camacho-Alonso, F., Jiménez-Torres, M. J., Orduña-Domingo, A., Gómez-García, F. Topical curcumin for the healing of carbon dioxide laser skin wounds in mice. *Photomed. Laser Surg.,* 2011, 29, 809-14.

[293] Gopinath, D., Ahmed, M. R., Gomathi, K., Chitra, K., Sehgal, P. K., Jayakumar, R. Dermal wound healing processes with curcumin incorporated collagen films. *Biomaterials*, 2004, 25, 1911-7.

[294] Chereddy, K. K., Coco, R., Memvanga, P. B., Ucakar, B., des Rieux, A., Vandermeulen, G., Préat, V. Combined effect of PLGA and curcumin on wound healing activity. *J. Control Release*, 2013, 171, 208-15.

[295] Gong, C., Wu, Q., Wang, Y., Zhang, D., Luo, F., Zhao, X., Wei, Y., Qian, Z. A biodegradable hydrogel system containing curcumin encapsulated in micelles for cutaneous wound healing. *Biomaterials*, 2013, 34, 6377-87.

[296] Mohanty, C., Das, M., Sahoo, S. K. Sustained wound healing activity of curcumin loaded oleic acid based polymeric bandage in a rat model. *Mol. Pharm.*, 2012, 9, 2801-11.

[297] Dai, M., Zheng, X., Xu, X., Kong, X., Li, X., Guo, G., Luo, F., Zhao, X., Wei, Y. Q., Qian, Z. Chitosan-alginate sponge: preparation and application in curcumin delivery for dermal wound healing in rat. *J. Biomed. Biotechnol.*, 2009, 2009, 595126. doi: 10.1155/2009/595126.

[298] Kaur, N., Garg, T., Goyal, A. K., Rath, G. Formulation, optimization and evaluation of curcumin-ß-cyclodextrin-loaded sponge for effective drug delivery in thermal burns chemotherapy. *Drug Deliv.*, 2014, 1-10. doi: 10.3109/10717544.2014.963900.

[299] Li, X., Chen, S., Zhang, B., Li, M., Diao, K., Zhang, Z., Li, J., Xu, Y., Wang, X., Chen, H. *In situ* injectable nano-composite hydrogel composed of curcumin, N,O-carboxymethyl chitosan and oxidized alginate for wound healing application. *Int. J. Pharm.*, 2012, 437, 110-9.

[300] Fu, S. Z., Meng, X. H., Fan, J., Yang, L. L., Wen, Q. L., Ye, S. J., Lin, S., Wang, B. Q., Chen, L. L., Wu, J. B., Chen, Y., Fan, J. M., Li, Z. Acceleration of dermal wound healing by using electrospun curcumin-loaded poly(ε-caprolactone)-poly(ethylene glycol)-poly(ε-caprolactone) fibrous mats. *J. Biomed. Mater. Res. B Appl. Biomater.*, 2014, 102, 533-42.

[301] Castangia, I., Nácher, A., Caddeo, C., Valenti, D., Fadda, A. M., Díez-Sales, O., Ruiz-Saurí, A., Manconi, M. Fabrication of quercetin and curcumin bionanovesicles for the prevention and rapid regeneration of full-thickness skin defects on mice. *Acta Biomater.*, 2014, 10, 1292-300.

[302] Satoskar, R. R., Shah, S. J., Shenoy, S. G. Evaluation of anti-inflammatory property of curcumin (diferuloyl methane) in patients with postoperative inflammation. *Int. J. Clin. Pharmacol. Ther. Toxicol.,* 1986, 24, 651-4.

[303] Chainani-Wu, N. Safety and anti-inflammatory activity of curcumin: a component of tumeric (*Curcuma longa*). *J. Altern. Complement. Med.*, 2003, 9, 161-8.

[304] Huang, M. T., Lysz, T., Ferraro, T., Abidi, T. F., Laskin, J. D., Conney, A. H. Inhibitory effects of curcumin on *in vitro* lipoxygenase and cyclooxygenase activities in mouse epidermis. *Cancer Res.*, 1991, 51, 813-9.

[305] Srivastava, K. C., Bordia, A., Verma, S. K. Curcumin, a major component of food spice turmeric (*Curcuma longa*) inhibits aggregation

and alters eicosanoid metabolism in human blood platelets. *Prostaglandins Leukot. Essent. Fatty Acids,* 1995, 52, 223-7.

[306] Shah, B. H., Nawaz, Z., Pertani, S. A., Roomi, A., Mahmood, H., Saeed, S. A., Gilani, A. H. Inhibitory effect of curcumin, a food spice from turmeric, on platelet-activating factor- and arachidonic acid-mediated platelet aggregation through inhibition of thromboxane formation and Ca2+ signaling. *Biochem. Pharmacol.*, 1999, 58, 1167-72.

[307] Hong, J., Bose, M., Ju, J., Ryu, J. H., Chen, X., Sang, S., Lee, M. J., Yang, C. S. Modulation of acrachidonic acid metabolism by curcumin and related beta-diketone derivatives: effects on cytosolic phospholipase A(2), cyclooxygenases and 5-lipoxygenase. *Carcinogenesis,* 2004, 25, 1671-9.

[308] Chun, K. S., Keum, Y. S., Han, S. S., Song, Y. S., Kim, S. H., Surh, Y. J. Curcumin inhibits phorbol ester-induced expression of cyclooxygenase-2 in mouse skin through suppression of extracellular signal-regulated kinase activity and NF-kappaB activation. *Carcinogenesis,* 2003, 24, 1515-24.

[309] Kim, G. Y., Kim, R. H., Lee, S. H., Yoon, M. S., Lee, H. J., Moon, D. O., Lee, C. M., Ahn, S. C., Park, Y. C., Park, Y. M. Curcumin inhibits immunostimulatory function of dendritic cells: MAPKs and translocation of NF-kappa B as potential targets. *J. Immunol.*, 2005, 174, 8116-24.

[310] Flynn, D. L., Rafferty, M. F., Boctor, A. M. Inhibition of 5-hydroxy-eicosatetraenoic acid (5-HETE) formation in intact human neutrophils by naturally-occurring diarylheptanoids: Inhibitory activities of curcuminoids and yakuchinones. *Prostaglandins Leukot. Med.*, 1986, 22, 357-60.

[311] Lee, J. H., Kim, J. W., Ko, N. Y., Mun, S. H., Her, E., Kim, B. K., Han, J. W., Lee, H. Y., Beaven, M. A., Kim, Y. M., Choi, W. S. Curcumin, a constituent of curry, suppresses IgE-mediated allergic response and mast cell activation at the level of Syk. *J. Allergy Clin. Immunol.*, 2008, 121, 1225-31.

[312] Suzuki, M., Nakamura, T., Iyoki, S., Fujiwara, A., Watanabe, Y., Mohri, K., Isobe, K., Ono, K., Yano, S. Elucidation of anti-allergic activities of curcumin-related compounds with a special reference to their anti-oxidative activities. *Biol. Pharm. Bull.*, 2005, 28, 1438-43.

[313] Kant, V., Gopal, A., Pathak, N. N., Kumar, P., Tandan, S. K., Kumar, D. Antioxidant and anti-inflammatory potential of curcumin accelerated the

cutaneous wound healing in streptozotocin-induced diabetic rats. *Int. Immunopharmacol.*, 2014, 20, 322-30.

[314] Gupta, B., Ghosh, B. *Curcuma longa* inhibits TNF-alpha induced expression of adhesion molecules on human umbilical vein endothelial cells. *Int. J. Immunopharmacol.*, 1999, 21, 745-57.

[315] Jia, S., Xie, P., Hong, S. J., Galiano, R., Singer, A., Clark, R. A., Mustoe, T. A. Intravenous curcumin efficacy on healing and scar formation in rabbit ear wounds under non-ischemic, ischemic, and ischemia-reperfusion conditions. *Wound Repair Regen.*, 2014. doi:10. 1111/wrr.12231.

[316] Murrell, J. G., McLaughlin, S. W., Tie, L., Laurencin, C. T., Chen, A. F., Nair, L. S. Curcumin-loaded poly(epsilon-caprolactone) nanofibres: diabetic wound dressing with anti-oxidant and anti-inflammatory properties. *Clin. Exp. Pharmacol. Physiol.,* 2009, 36, 1149-56.

[317] Abe, Y., Hashimoto, S., Horie, T. Curcumin inhibition of inflammatory cytokine production by human peripheral blood monocytes and alveolar macrophages. *Pharmacol. Res.*, 1999, 39, 41-7.

[318] Kang, B. Y., Chung, S. W., Chung, W., Im, S., Hwang, S. Y., Kim, T. S. Inhibition of interleukin-12 production in lipopolysaccharide-activated macrophages by curcumin. *Eur. J. Pharmacol.,* 1999, 384, 191-5.

[319] Liu, J. Y., Lin, S. J., Lin, J. K. Inhibitory effects of curcumin on protein kinase C activity induced by 12-O-tetradecanoyl-phorbol-13-acetate in NIH 3T3 cells. *Carcinogenesis*, 1993, 14, 857-61.

[320] Jobin, C., Bradham, C. A., Russo, M. P., Juma, B., Narula, A. S., Brenner, D. A., Sartor, R. B. Curcumin blocks cytokine-mediated NF-kappa B activation and proinflammatory gene expression by inhibiting inhibitory factor I-kappa B kinase activity. *J. Immunol.*, 1999, 163, 3474-83.

[321] Jurenka, J. S. Anti-inflammatory properties of curcumin, a major constituent of *Curcuma longa*: a review of preclinical and clinical research. *Altern. Med. Rev.*, 2009, 14, 141-53.

[322] Joe, B., Lokesh, B. R. Effect of curcumin and capsaicin on arachidonic acid metabolism and lysosomal enzyme secretion by rat peritoneal macrophages. *Lipids,* 1997, 32, 1173-80.

[323] Kunchandy, E., Rao, M. N. A. Oxygen radical scavenging activity of curcumin. *Int. J. Pharm.*, 1990, 58, 237-40.

[324] Panchatcharam, M., Miriyala, S., Gayathri, V. S., Suguna, L. Curcumin improves wound healing by modulating collagen and decreasing reactive oxygen species. *Mol. Cell. Biochem.*, 2006, 290, 87-96.

[325] Pendurthi, U. R., Williams, J. T., Rao, L. V. Inhibition of tissue factor gene activation in cultured endothelial cells by curcumin. Suppression of activation of transcription factors Egr-1, AP-1 and NF-kappa B. *Arterioscler. Thromb. Vas. Biol.,* 1997, 17, 3406-13.

[326] Bierhaus, A., Zhang, Y., Quehenberger, P., Luther, T., Haase, M., Muller, M., Mackman, N., Ziegler, R., Nawroth, P. P. The dietary pigment curcumin reduces endothelial tissue factor gene expression by inhibiting binding of AP-1 to the DNA and activation of NF-kappa B. *Thromb. Haemost.,* 1997, 77, 772-82.

[327] Thaloor, D., Singh, A. K., Sidhu, G. S., Prasad, P. V., Kleinman, H. K., Maheshwari, R. K. Inhibition of angiogenic differentiation of human umbilical vein endothelial cells by curcumin. *Cell Growth Differ.,* 1998, 9, 305-12.

[328] Arbiser, J. L., Klauber, N., Rohan, R., van Leeuwen, R., Huang, M. T., Fisher, C., Flynn, E., Byers, H. R. Curcumin is *an in vivo* inhibitor of angiogenesis. *Mol. Med.*, 1998, 4, 376-83.

[329] Kiran, M. S., Kumar, V. B., Viji, R. I., Sherin, G. T., Rajasekharan, K. N., Sudhakaran, P. R. Opposing effects of curcuminoids on serum stimulated and unstimulated angiogenic response. *J. Cell. Physiol.*, 2008, 215, 251-64.

[330] Phan, T. T., See, P., Lee, S. T., Chan, S. Y. Protective effects of curcumin against oxidative damage on skin cells *in vitro*: its implication for wound healing. *J. Trauma*, 2001, 51, 927-31.

[331] Mani, H., Sidhu, G. S., Kumari, R., Gaddipati, J. P., Seth, P., Maheshwari, R. K. Curcumin differentially regulates TGF-beta1, its receptors and nitric oxide synthase during impaired wound healing. *Biofactors,* 2002, 16, 29-43.

[332] Madhyastha, R., Madhyastha, H., Nakajima, Y., Omura, S., Maruyama, M. Curcumin facilitates fibrinolysis and cellular migration during wound healing by modulating urokinase plasminogen activator expression. *Pathophysiol. Haemost. Thromb.*, 2010, 37, 59-66.

[333] Scharstuhl, A., Mutsaers, H. A., Pennings, S. W., Szarek, W. A., Russel, F. G., Wagener, F. A. Curcumin-induced fibroblast apoptosis and *in vitro* wound contraction are regulated by antioxidants and heme oxygenase: implications for scar formation. *J. Cell. Mol. Med.*, 2009, 13, 712-25.

[334] Kang, J. Y., Huang, H., Zhu, F. Q. Effect of curcumin on growth and function of fibroblast in human hyperplastic scar. *Zhongguo Zhong Xi Yi Jie He Za Zhi*, 2009, 29, 1100-3.

[335] Schraufstatter, E., Bernt, H. Antibacterial action of curcumin and related compounds. *Nature*, 1949, 164, 456-7.

[336] Neelofar, K., Shreaz, S., Rimple, B., Muralidhar, S., Nikhat, M., Khan, L. A. Curcumin as a promising anticandidal of clinical interest. *Can. J. Microbiol.*, 2011, 57, 204-10.

[337] Zandi, K., Ramedani, E., Mohammadi, K., Tajbakhsh, S., Deilami, I., Rastian, Z., Fouladvand, M., Yousefi, F., Farshadpour, F. Evaluation of antiviral activities of curcumin derivative against HSV-1 in Vero cell line. *Nat. Prod. Commun.*, 2010, 5, 1935-8.

[338] Si, X., Wang, Y., Wong, J., Zhang, J., McManus, B. M., Luo, H. Dysregulation of the ubiquitin-proteasome system by curcumin suppresses coxsackievirus B3 replication. *J. Virol.*, 2007, 81, 3142-50.

[339] Krausz, A. E., Adler, B. L., Cabral, V., Navati, M., Doerner, J., Charafeddine, R., Chandra, D., Liang, H., Gunther, L., Clendaniel, A., Harper, S., Friedman, J. M., Nosanchuk, J. D., Friedman, A. J. Curcumin-encapsulated nanoparticles as innovative antimicrobial and wound healing agent. *Nanomedicine*, 2014, pii: S1549-9634(14)00527-9. doi:10.1016/j.nano.2014.09.004.

[340] Jones, M. K., Wang, H., Peskar, B. M., Levin, E., Itani, R. M., Sarfeh, I. J., Tarnawski, A. S. Inhibition of angiogenesis by nonsteroidal anti-inflammatory drugs: insight into mechanisms and implications for cancer growth and ulcer healing. *Nat. Med.*, 1999, 5, 1418-23.

[341] Braiman-Wiksman, L., Solomonik, I., Spira, R., Tennenbaum, T. Novel insights into wound healing sequence of events. *Toxicol. Pathol.*, 2007, 35, 767-79.

In: Chinese Herbs and Herbal Medicine
Editor: Brian L. Duke
ISBN: 978-1-63482-085-1
© 2015 Nova Science Publishers, Inc.

Chapter II

Chinese Medicinal Herb: A Clinical Monograph of Radix Bupleuri (Chai Hu)

Angela Wei Hong Yang and Jenny Kreiner
Discipline of Chinese Medicine, School of Health Sciences, RMIT University

Abstract

Radix Bupleuri (Chai Hu) is one of the most commonly used herbs in the Chinese medicine clinical practice. In Chinese medicine, it is believed that Radix Bupleuri (Chai Hu) is acrid, cool and bitter and enters Liver and Gallbladder meridians. It is used to reduce fever, release the stagnation of Liver Qi and raise clear Yang. Details of its actions, indications, contraindications, dosage and control are discussed from Chinese medicine perspective. In Western medicine, the clinical and experimental studies have shown that Radix Bupleuri (Chai Hu) has anti-inflammatory, antimicrobial, antiviral, immune-regulatory and anti-tumour effects. Radix Bupleuri (Chai Hu) also has effects on central nervous system, cardiovascular system, digestive system and metabolism. This monograph presents details of its pharmacodynamics, pharmacokinetics and mechanism, toxicology and interactions as well as side effects with evidence from comprehensive literature search.

Guidelines for its use and regulatory control in different countries are also reviewed.

Keywords: Radix Bupleuri, Chinese Thorowax root, Bupleurum, Hare's ear root, Chinese thoroughwax, Shrubby hare's ear, Sickle-leaf hare's ear, Thoroughwax, Saiko, Siho, Chai Cao, Di Xun, Ru Cao, Shan Cai, Zi Hu, Nan Hu, Ya Hu

Introduction

Radix Bupleuri (Chai Hu) is a commonly used herb in Chinese medicine in China, Japan, Asia Pacific as well as in western countries such as Europe, USA and Australia. It was originally called "Zi Hu (茈胡)" and described in Shennong's Classic of Materia Medica (*Shennong Ben Cao Jing*) [1, 2]. The dried root or dried whole herb is used for its therapeutic effects. Its flavour is acrid and bitter and it is cool in nature. Radix Bupleuri (Chai Hu) has been used for thousands of years to enter Liver and Gallbladder meridians to reduce fever, release the stagnation of Liver Qi and raise clear Yang. It is used for common cold, menstrual disorders, pain in chest, epigastric and hypochondriac regions, and prolapsed of the uterine or anal and diarrhoea due to collapse of Spleen Qi [1, 3-5].

Species

The root of nineteen species [1, 5-9] and the whole herb of 7 species [6] are used for medicinal purposes, including *Bupleurum chinense* DC. (Bei Chai Hu, 北柴胡) [1, 9], *Bupleurum scorzonerifolium* Willd. (Nan Chai Hu, 南柴胡) [1, 9], *Bupleurum angustissimum* (Franch.) kitag (Xian Ye Chai Hu, 线叶柴胡) [6], *Bupleurum aureum* Fisch. (Jin Huang Chai Hu, 金黄柴胡) [6], *Bupleurum bicaule* Helm. (Zhui Ye Chai Hu, 锥叶柴胡) [6], *Bupleurum chaishoui* Shan et Sheh (Chai Shou, 柴首) [6], *Bupleurum densiflorum* Rupr. (Mi Hua Chai Hu, 密花柴胡) [6], *Bupleurum exaltatum Marsh.* Bieb. (Xin Jiang Chai Hu, 新疆柴胡) [6], *Bupleurum falcatum* L. [10], *Bupleurum komarovianum* Lincz. (Chang Bai Chai Hu, 长白柴胡) [6], *Bupleurum marginatum* Wall. ex DC. (Zhu Ye Chai Hu, 竹叶柴胡) [6], *Bupleurum marginatum* Wall. ex DC. var. stenophyllum (Wolff) Shan et Y. Li (Zhai Zhu Ye Chai Hu, 窄竹叶柴) [6], *Bupleurum rotundifolium* L.(Yuan Ye Chai Hu, 圆叶柴胡) [6], *Bupleurum rigidum* [7], *Bupleurum salicifolium* Soland [8], *Bupleurum sibiricum* Vest (Xing An Chai Hu, 兴安柴胡) [6], *Bupleurum smithii* Wolff var. parvifolium Shan et Y. Li (Xiao Ye Hei Cahi Hu, 小叶黑柴胡) [6], *Bupleurum triradiatum* Adams ex Hoffm. (San Fu Chai Hu, 三辐柴胡) [6], *Bupleurum yinchowense* Shan et Y. Li (Yin Zhou Chai Hu, 银州柴胡) [6], *Bupleurum hamiltoni* Balak. (B. tenue Buch. Ham. ex D. Don) (Xiao Chai Hu, 小柴胡) [6], *Bupleurum longicaule* Wall. ex DC. var. franchetii de Boiss. (Kong Xin Chai Hu, 空心柴胡) [6], *Bupleurum longicaule* Wall. ex DC. var. giraldii Wolff (Qin Ling Chai Hu, 秦岭柴胡) [6], *Bupleurum malconense* Shan et Y. Li (Ma Er Kang Chai Hu, 马尔康柴胡) [6], *Bupleurum microcephalum* Diels (Ma Wei Chai Hu, 马尾柴胡) [6], *Bupleurum tianshanicum* Freyn (Tian Shan Chai Hu, 天山柴胡) [6], and *Bupleurum wenchuanense* Shan et Y. Li (Wen Zhou Chai Hu, 汶州柴胡) [6]. Among them, *Bupleurum chinense* DC. (Bei Chai Hu) and *Bupleurum scorzonerifolium* Willd. (Nan Chai Hu) are the two main species.

Chemical Constituents

A total of ninety-six chemical constituents are isolated from *Bupleurum chinense* DC. (Bei Chai Hu) and thirty-two chemical constituents are identified from *Bupleurum scorzonerifolium* Willd. (Nan Chai Hu), including Δ^{22}-Stigmasterol [11, 12], δ-Cadinene [11], α-Copaene [12], α-Cubebene [11, 12], γ-Decalactone [6, 12], (E)-geranyl acetone [11], β-Fenchene [11, 12], γ-Heptalactone [6], α-Longipinene [12], o-Methoxy phenol [6, 12], γ-Octalactone [6], γ-Rudecalactone [12], α-Spinasterol [2, 6, 12], β-Terpinene [11, 12], α-Terpineol [11, 12], β-Terpineol [11], γ-undecalactone [6], 11α-methoxyosaikosaponin f [4], 2-Heptenoic acid [6, 12], 2-Methyl cyclopentanone [11, 12], 2-Nonenoic acid [6, 12], 2-Octenoic acid [6, 12], 3''-O-Acetyl saikosaponin a [4, 12], 3''-O-Acetyl saikosaponin b_4 [4], 3''-O-Acetyl saikosaponin d [4], 6''-O-Acetyl saikosaponin a [2, 4], 6''-O-Acetyl saikosaponin d [4], Adonitol [6, 12], Aromadendrene [11, 12], Bupleurum polysaccharide [13], Bupleurumol [1, 12], Camphene [11, 12], Caproic acid [12], Carvacrone [11], Carveol [11], Carvone [12], Caryophyllene [11],

Chikusaikoside I [4], Chikusaikoside II [4], cis-β-Terpineol [12], Cresol [6], Daikogenin [1], Ethylohenol [6], Eugenol [6, 12], Geraniol [11], Heptanoic acid [6, 12], Hexadecanoic acid [6, 12], Hexahydrofarnesyl acetone [11], Hexanoic acid [11], Humulene [11, 12], Isopsoralen [12], Kaempferitrin [12, 14], Kaempferol [14], Kaempferol-3-O-α-L-arabinopyranoside-7-O-α-L-rhamnopyranoside [14], Kaempferol-7-rhamnoside [14], Ledol [11, 12], Lignoceric acid [12], Limonene [2, 11, 12], Linalool [11, 12], Linolenic acid [12], Longifolene [11, 12], Longispinogenin [12], Messoia lactone [6], Myrcene [2, 11, 12], Myrtenol [2, 11], Nonanoic acid [6], Nootkatone [11, 12], n-Tridecane [11, 12], Octanoic acid [6], Oleic acid [1], Palmitic acid [12], Patchoulane [11, 12], Pelargonic acid [12], Pentanoic acid [6, 12], Petroselic acid [12], Phenol [6, 12], Pulegone [11, 12], Rutin [1, 6], Saikogenin E [12], Saikogenin F [12], Saikogenin G [12], Saikosaponin a [2, 4, 12, 15-17], Saikosaponin b_1 [4], Saikosaponin b_2 [4], Saikosaponin b_3 [2, 4], Saikosaponin b_4 [2, 4], Saikosaponin c [2, 4, 6, 12, 16, 18], Saikosaponin d [4, 15], osaponin d [2, 4, 12, 15-17], osaponin e [2, 4], osaponin f [2, 4], Saikosaponin s_1 [12, 16], Saikosaponin t [12], Saikosaponin V [12], Stearic acid [12], Stigmasterol [12], Thymol [6, 12], trans-β-Terpineol [12], Vanillin acetate [6, 12], Volatile oil [18], β-Elemene [11], α-Farnesene [11], γ-Muurolene [11], Isoborneol [11], Isoquercetin [1, 6], Isorhamnetin [1, 6], Kaempferol-7-rhamnoside [6], Narcissin [1, 6], and Quercetin [1, 6].

No toxic constituents identified are related to *Bupleurum chinense* DC. (Bei Chai Hu) or *Bupleurum scorzonerifolium* Willd. (Nan Chai Hu) Only the dried root of *Bupleurum longiradiatum* Turcz. (Da Ye Chai Hu) is highly toxic and should not be used for medicinal purposes. Toxic constituents that have been isolated and identified are bupleurotoxin, bupleuonol, acetyl-bupleurotoxin and bupleurynol [4].

Spectroscopy and multivariate data analysis were applied to sixty-seven Radix Bupleuri (Chai Hu) samples to discriminate *Bupleurum chinense* DC. (Bei Chai Hu) or *Bupleurum scorzonerifolium* Willd. (Nan Chai Hu), and explored the influences of habitat and culture method on the quality of Radix Bupleuri (Chai Hu) based on their metabolomics profiles. Higher levels of arginine, citric acid, sucrose, Saikosaponin b_1/b_2 analogs, volatile oil with an (E)-2-olefin aldehyde fragment, and fatty acids were detected in *Bupleurum scornerifolium*, and more Saikosaponins a/c/d analogs in *Bupleurum chinense* DC. Higher amount of *Saikosaponins* a/c/d were found in samples yielded from Shaanxi and lipids in samples from Shanxi province [19]. No obvious difference was detected between cultivars and wild type. Studies on morphological features of the Bupleurum also showed that it contained different *Saikosaponins yield*. The roots of *Bupleurum scorzonerifolium* and *Bupleurum falcatum*, the cork cell of the cork cambium contained much higher contents of *Saikosaponins* a, c and d than did the cortex; while in the root of *Bupleurum chinense* DC., the cortex contained higher contents of Saikosaponins a, c and d than the cork [20].

Mechanisms of Action

Radix Bupleuri (Chai Hu) have been reported to have anti-inflammatory, anti-microbial, anti-viral, and immune-regulatory effects, as well as effects on central nervous system (including anti-pyretic, sedative, analgesic, anti-neural and memory impairment, anti-epileptic and antitussive effects), cardiovascular system, and digestive system. It has anti-tumour effects. It also has a regulatory effect on the metabolism and other systems.

Anti-Inflammatory Effects

Essential oils extracts from *Bupleurum chinense* DC. [21], *Bupleurum fruitcesens* [22] and *Bupleurum fruitcosum* [23] have exerted anti-inflammatory effects on mouse oedema induced by carrageenin. When induced by prostaglandin E_1 (PGE_1), the essential oil of *Bupleurum fruitcescens* [22] also has an anti-inflammatory on rat oedema. Anti-inflammatory effects have proven to be active when induced by tetradecanoylphorbol acetate on mouse oedema by extracts from *Bupleurum fruitcesens* including fruitcesaponins A, B and C [24]. Swellings of the rats were proven to be inhibited when implanting a piece of cotton wool with extracts of essential oil from *Bupleurum fruitcosum* [23]. One study highlighted the outcome of using essential oil extract by formulating an intranasal delivery system in an aqueous solution used in the form of nasal spray [25], proved to have an effect on rising body temperature on rabbits and rats. It has also an effect on poliomyelitis in guinea pigs [26].

The similar components of the essential oil were identified in the extract of the aboveground and the root of *Bupleurum malconense* as well as the root of *Bupleurum chinense DC*. An active component of anti-inflammatory and analgesic, caryophyllene oxide was detected in high content. This suggested that as a local substitute, *Bupleurum malconense* has a certain scientific basis of the treatment for cold and fever [27].

Radix Bupleuri (Chai Hu) were discovered to have no protective effect against histamine induced or anaphylactoid shock [1, 28]. This experiment indicated that injection of Radix Bupleuri (Chai Hu) had no significant inhibition on the increase of capillary permeability in rabbits with intravenous administration or on rat scale-induced paw swelling with intraperitoneal administration [29]. On the contrary, one recent study showed that Saikosaponin a and Saikosaponin d exhibited significant anti-inflammatory activity in two different murine models of acute inflammation, carrageenin-induced paw oedema in rats and acetic acid-induced vascular permeability in mice. Saikosaponin a and Saikosaponin d demonstrated potent anti-inflammatory activity through inhibitory effects on NF-κB activation and thereby on inducible nitric-oxide synthase (iNOS), cyclooxygenase (COX)-2 and pro-inflammatory cytokines [30]. Hence, Saikosaponins have considerable effects on the inflammatory process by inhibiting the expression of iNOS and COX-2, suppressing major pro- inflammatory cytokines such as the tumour necrosis factor-α (TNF-α) and interleukin (IL)-6 [30-32], including exudation, capillary permeability, inflammatory media release, leukocyte migration and connective tissue proliferation [31, 33].

Polysaccharides have been studied extensively and found to have immunomodulatory effects on inflammation. Complementary cascade, pro-inflammatory mediators, cytokines and chemokines all contribute to inflammatory responses. Polysaccharides BC-PS_2 was isolated from the root of *Bupleurum chinense* DC. as an anti-complementary agent in one study. It was identified as a branched polysaccharide and which inhibited the excessive complementary cascade. Bioassay experiments revealed that BC-PS2 inhibited activation on both the classical and the alternative pathway. Preliminary studies indicated that polysaccharides interacted with C_{1q}, C_2 and C_9 components of the activation pathway [34].

Crude polysaccharides isolated from the roots of *Bupleurum smithii* var. parvifolium initiated anti-complementary activity and regulated immunomodulatory functions on macrophages. Enhanced murine peritoneal macrophages were detected *in vivo* study. Treatment with polysaccharides was found to have up-regulated phagocytic functions of macrophages and inhibited lipopolysaccharides (LPS)-induced productions of nitric oxide and pro-inflammatory cytokines (IL-1β, IL-6 and tumour necrosis factor- α) [35, 36]. Significant increases in splenic index, percentage of phagocytosis and phagocytic index in macrophacocytes in the abdominal cavities were detected when intraperitoneal injections of polysaccharides were administered in mice [35, 37] as well as increased indexes of the macrophacocytes in the serum neutralising antibody titer of influenza viruses, the transformation rate of splenic lymph cells and the activity of natural killer cells. Bupleurum polysaccharides have been found to have up-regulated phagocytic activities but inhibited LPS-induced productions of pro-inflammatory mediators [35].

Polysaccharides from *Bupleurum chinense* DC. were detected to significantly impair the leukocyte infiltration and relieve lung injury in mice with LPS-induced acute pneumonia. Lung reperfusion injury and haemorrhagic shock was induced in mice subjects. Crude polysaccharides isolated from the roots of *Bupleurum smithii var. parvifolium* were administered orally and they ameliorated pathological injury with lessened complement C3c deposit in lung, reduced leukocytes, fluid protein concentration and lung myeloperioxidase. Total haemolytic activity and decreased cyctokines activity were observed [38].

P-selectin has been considered as a promising target for therapeutics of acute inflammatory-related diseases. P-selectin-mediated adhesion between endothelium and neutrophils is a crucial process leading to acute inflammatory injury. In one study, water-soluble polysaccharides isolated from *Bupleurum chinense* DC. was evaluated for its therapeutical effects on acute inflammatory injury and antagonistic function against P-selectin-mediated neutrophils adhesion. Results indicated that polysaccharides significantly impaired the leukocyte infiltration and relieved lung injury in LPS-induced acute pneumonia model. It also significantly blocked the binding of P-selectin to neutrophils and inhibited P-selectin-mediated neutrophils rolling along CHO-P cell monolayer. *In vitro* protein binding assay showed direct evidence indicating that polysaccarides-treatment significantly eliminated the interactions between rhP-Fc and its physiological ligand PSGL-1 at protein level. These results provide a novel therapeutic strategy for amelioration of inflammation-related disease processes by polysaccharides from *Bupleurum chinense* DC [39].

Prostaglandin E_2 (PGE_2), an important lipid inflammatory mediator, was found in a study to be inhibited by Bupleurum injection. Hypothalamic neurocytes were cultured *in vitro*, added with rrIL-1β (a recombinant cytokine) stimulation and then with different concentrations of Bupleurum injection. Bupleurum injections significantly inhibited the rate of PGE_2 *in vitro* cultured hypothalamic neurocytes. This evidence highlighted that Radix Bupleuri (Chai Hu) concentration had an inhibitory effect of PGE_2 inflammatory mediator [40].

Bupleurum polysaccharides, isolated from *Bupleurum smithii var. parvifolium*, possessed immunomodulatory activity, particularly on inflammation. Bacterial endotoxin LPS triggered innate immune responses through toll-like receptor 4 on host cell membrane. This study indicated that therapeutic effects of Bupleurum polysaccharides on suppression of LPS's pathogenecity could be associated with the modulating of toll-like receptor 4 signalling pathway [41].

A study administered a Chinese herbal formula, Xiao Chai Hu Tang (Shosaiko-to in Japanese) with Radix Bupleuri (Chai Hu) as the chief herb, to induce interferon (IFN) in mice. It indicated that pre-treatment of Xiao Chai Hu Tang was able to suppress IFN and induce IFN when administered. Moreover, evidence also further showed that spleen cells from untreated mice could also produce IFN when they were cultured with Xiao Chai Hu Tang. Additionally, serum IFN was also induced by the adoptive transfer of spleen cells from Xiao Chai Hu Tang treated mice to normal mice. On the other hand, oral administration of Xiao Chai Hu Tang also induced IFN-α/β in the serum. While IFN activity induced by intraperitoneal injection administration of Xiao Chai Hu Tang declined after repeated treatments, the activity induced by oral administration did not decline during a long-term treatment. These results demonstrated that Xiao Chai Hu Tang is an IFN-α/β inducer capable of repeated oral administration [42].

Anti-Microbial and Anti-Viral Effects

Polyacetlene is a secondary bioactive metabolite found in Bupleuri genus. It had significant antibiotic effects on Gram positive bacteria, *Staphylococcus aureus* and *Bacillus subtilis* [8] with the isolation of 8S-heptadeca-2(Z), 9(Z)-diene-4,6-diyne-1,8-diol from *Bupleurum salicifolium* Soland. However, one experiment revealed that intravenous injection of Radix Bupleuri (Chai Hu) had no significant inhibition on Staphylococcus albus, Diplocaccus of Neisser, Diplococcus pneumoniae, Streptococcus hemoliticus, or Pseudomonas pyocyanea. There is only slight inhibition on Staphylococcus aureus with the paper strip method [29].

IFN expression has been discovered when a Bupleurum dominant Chinese herbal formula was tested on Coxsackievirus B 1 (CVB1). CVB1 infection is known to cause high morbidity and mortality in children; however, there is no effective drug for treating this disease. One study examined the antiviral activity of Xiao Chai Hu Tang, against CVB1 infection and its mechanisms of action. Findings indicated that Xiao Chai Hu Tang neutralised the CVB1-induced cytopathic effect in human neonatal foreskin fibroblast cell line [43]. The time-of-addition studies showed that Xiao Chai Hu (50, 100 and 200 μg/ml) added at various time of pre-infection (-1 to -3 hour), co-infection (0 hour) and post-infection (1 approximately 3 hours) could inhibit CVB1 infection. Interestingly, Xiao Chai Hu Tang also showed an inhibition on viral replication through the induction of IFN-α/β expression. This study revealed that Radix Bupleuri (Chai Hu) might interfere the early stage of viral replication (prophylactic effect) and viral replication after infection (therapeutic effect) through the induction of Type 1 IFN expression [43].

Intravenous injection of *Bupleurum chinense* DC. which contain active constituents of Saikosaponin a, exhibited strong inhibition on influenza viruses *in vitro* [33]. However, one experiment highlighted that it did not inhibit A_3 type of influenza virus in chicken embryo allantoic cavities [29]. Xiao Chai Hu Tang inhibited human immunodeficiency virus (HIV) type 1 replication at a concentration of 25 μg/ml *in vitro* [44]. One recent study screened the antiviral agents from *Bupleurum rigidum* and *Scrophularia scorodonia* medicinal plants. Three Saikosaponins, seven iridoids and one phenylpropanoid glycoside were tested *in vitro* against herpes simplex virus type 1 (HSV-1), vesicular stomatitis virus [45], and poliovirus type 1. Five of these compounds showed the antiviral activity against vesicular stomatitis virus. None of the Saikosaponins were active against HSV-1, but the iridoid scorodioside showed moderate *in vitro* anti-HSV-1 activity (30.6 % at 500 μg/ml) [46].

A study also demonstrated that simultaneous intramuscular administration of injection of Radix Bupleurum (Chai Hu) including eye drops with 10% dilution had an effect on herpes simplex keratitis and sub-bulbar conjunctiva [29].

Immuno-Regulatory Effects

Saikosaponin d from *Bupleurum falcatum* L. could stimulate immunological lymphocyte actions *in vivo*. A significant increase in the numbers of the immunoglobulin (Ig) M plague forming in mice with sheep red blood cells enhanced splenic cell proliferation responses to the stimulation of T and B-cell both before and after immunisation of Saikosaponin d extract. Increased spread of microphages and lysosomal enzyme activity, improved chemiluminenses of the macrophages and IL-1 production were also detected

[47]. Saikosaponin d bi-directionally controlled the growth of T lymphocyte response stimulated by concanavalin A, anti CD_3, monoclonal antibody and calcium ionophore A23187 plus phorbol 12-myristate 13 acetate. It also regulated the responses to suboptimum stimuli of agnoists, promoted IL-2 production and IL-2 receptor expression and accelerated c-fos gene transcription [48]. On human lymphocytes, Bupleurum-containing compounds were found to induce the secretion of granulocyte-macrophage colony-stimulating factor in a dose dependent manner [49]. However, some animal experiments demonstrated that the decoction of Radix Bupleuri (Chai Hu) and Saikosaponins decreased the functions of the immune system by inhibiting the thymus function [6].

Polysaccharide, bupleuran 2IIc, extracted from the roots of *Bupleurum falcatum* L. on IL-6 was investigated in order to clarify the mechanism of enhanced immunoglobulin secretion from B cells. Bupleuran 2IIc stimulated B cells. IL-6 secretion and the transcription of IL-6 mRNA activities were also enhanced. Results suggest that bupleuran 2IIc stimulated the secretion of IL-6 as the active site, and it may partially contribute to the enhancement of IgM secretion as an autocrine and/or paracrine mechanism [50]. One study investigated that crude polysaccharides isolated from the roots of *Bupleurum smithii var. parvifolium*, had beneficial effects on autoimmune disease induced by Campylobacter jejuni in BALB/c mice. This *in vitro* study showed that treatment with *Bupleurum* polysaccharides protected kidneys from glomerular injury with reduced immunoglobulin deposition and lowered proteinuria, along with increased production of serum autoantibodies and total IgG was also inhibited. Positive signs also included improved weight loss and reduced spleen swelling [51]. These findings suggested that *Bupleurum* polysaccharides had a beneficial effect on systemic lupus erythematosus-like syndrome [51].

The glycone moiety of Saikosaponin a exhibited its capability of attaching a carrier protein in the preparation for immunogen for Saikosaponin–specific enzyme-linked immunoabsorbent assay (ELISA) in rabbits [52]. Lignin-like moiety was also detected in polyphenolic substances in *Bupleurum chinense* DC [53-55]. These were considered to be immunopharmacologically active substances. A wide range of mitogenic molecular activity to murine lymphoctyes was revealed with hot water extracts of Radix Bupleurum (Chai Hu) [53, 54].

Anti-Pyretic Effects

Chemical constituents with anti-pyretic effects identified were *Saikosaponins*, engenol, heanoic acid, γ-undecalactone, ρ-methooxy-acetonphenone and α-spinasterol [4]. Anti-pyretic effects were detected when extractions of these oil and saponin faction from *Bupleurum* when administered intraperitioneally in rats [29]. The manner of administration and dosage could have different impact on the fever. Intranasal spray had anti-pyretic effects on rabbits and rats [25]. Oral or intramuscular administration of a decoction of Radix Bupleuri (Chai Hu) could reduce fever induced by typhoid vaccine [56] or sour milk [57]. Another report indicated that when administered intravenously, the anti-pyretic effect in rabbits was not significant [29]. Formulation of an intranasal delivery system for the essential oil in an aqueous solution used in the form of nasal spray was also studied *in vivo* and developed. Radix Bupleuri (Chai Hu) essential oil extract was administered intranasal to rabbits with fever induced by subcutaneous injection of turpentine decreased body temperature markedly (0.5, 0.8 and 1.0 degrees C respectively at the dose of oil from 1, 2 and 4 g Bupleuri/body). In addition, the administration also significantly reduced fever in rats induced by intramuscular injection of Bupleuri essential oil. The findings suggested that the formulation of nasal spray for the essential oil from Radix Bupleuri could be potentially effective in the treatment of fever [25]. Further study examined a nasal *in situ* gel system for Radix Bupleuri (Chai Hu) employing gellan gum as a polymer. The anti-pyretic effect produced by *in situ* gel formulation was investigated in fevered rabbits and compared to an intranasal solution. Intranasal administration to fevered rabbits decreased body temperature markedly (1.1°C at the doses of oil from 1.5 g Bupleuri/body) and the effect could last for 20-30 hours. It showed that it could prolong the effective time up to 24 hours compared with 4-6 hours in Radix Bupleuri (Chai Hu) intranasal solution. Overall results suggested that Radix Bupleuri (Chai Hu) *in situ* gel had greater effectiveness than the solution in the treatment of fever [58, 59].

Sedative Effects

Saikosides comprising Saikosaponin fraction (500 mg/kg) and Saikosaoponin a, with the latter by means of intraperitoneal injection and the former orally administered, presented inhibition of excitement and decreased spontaneous activity of mice as well as lengthen sleep induced by hexabarbitol

[33]. Xiao Yao Wan is a Chinese herbal formula with the predominant herb Radix Bupleurum (Chai Hu) and commonly indicated for Liver stagnation and Spleen deficiency syndrome. Chromatography analysis of Xiao Yao Wan showed that there was an increase in plasma β-endorphin and dopamine while epinephrine decreased after the administration of Xiao Yao Wan in the experimental group, which indicated that Xiao Yao Wan could regulate nervous and endocrine systems and contribute to the improvement of patients with Liver stagnation and Spleen deficiency syndrome [60].

Analgesic Effects

Saponin fraction (478 mg/kg) derived from the root of *Bupleurum chinense* DC. was used in an *in vitro* study while electrical desiccation was used on the tails of rats, analgesic effect was observed [21]. When administered orally or intraperitoneally, Saikosaponin fraction also showed an analgesic effect in mice. One experiment showed intraperitoneal administration of Saikosaponin a with 50 and 100 mg/kg reduced acetic acid induced writhing in mice [4].

Anti-Neural and Memory Impairment Effects

Bupleurum falcatum L. is widely used in the treatment of various psychosomatic diseases in traditional Oriental medicine and it is considered as an effective therapeutic intervention for memory impairment. One study examined its effects on stress-induced alterations in learning and memory in rats using the Morris water maze and elevated plus maze behavioural tests. *Bupleurum falcatum* L. treatment on the cholinergic system indicated changes in neuronal choline acetyltransferase and acetylcholinesterase immunoreactivity in the hippocampus. The treatment produced a significant improvement in escape latency in the Morris water maze and generated an anxiolytic-like effect in the elevated plus maze. Consistent with the behavioural data, *Bupleurum falcatum* L. significantly attenuated the immobilisation stress-induced loss of cholinergic immunoreactivity in the hippocampus. These findings indicated that *Bupleurum falcatum* L. had a protective effect against repeated immobilisation stress-induced neuronal and cognitive impairments, and *Bupleurum falcatum* L. may be useful in the treatment of stress-induced memory impairment [61].

Anti-Epileptic Effects

Saikosaponin a, the main constituent of *Bupleurum chinense* DC., has demonstrated the anti-epileptic activity in several studies [62-67]. One study indicated that Saikosaponin a could inhibit N-methyl-D-aspartate (NMDA) (a molecular device responsible for controlling synaptic plasticity and memory function) receptor current and persistent sodium current [63]. This study highlighted the efficacy of Saikosaponin a effect in the suppression of spontaneous recurrent epileptiform discharges in acquired epilepsy models and continuous epileptiform high-frequency bursts in status epilepticus models. Another study found that Saikosaponin a significantly inhibited epileptiform discharges frequency and duration in hippocampal CA1 neurons in the 4AP seizure model in a dose-dependent manner. Accumulated data in this study indicated that Saikosaponin a was able to inhibit epileptiform discharges and contribute to the anticonvulsant mechanisms of Saikosaponin a [66]. In another study, intraabdominal injection of Bupleurum root on animal models and effect of Bupleurum root on the electroencephalogram (EEG) and hippocampal slice by electroencephalograph and glass microelectrode were observed extracellularly. Both the seizure time and duration of seizures were significantly shortened and the interval of seizure significantly prolonged [67]. These findings suggested that Saikosaponin a may be a potential anticonvulsant candidate for the clinical treatment of epilepsy [63].

Emetic Effects

Powder of *Bupleurum chinense* DC. (5 g /kg) or volatile oil (0.7 g/kg) from the root of *Bupleurum chinense* DC. did not produce emetic reactions in pigeons [21].

Antitussive Effects

Saikosasponin a was discovered to have a significant antitussive effect in a concentration-dependent manner. An experiment showed that when 9.1 mg/kg of Saikosaponin fraction was administered intraperitoneally in guniea pigs, this produced an equivalent antitussive effect to 7.6 mg/kg of codeine phosphate [33]. Dosage related Saikosaponin was most obvious with intraperitoneal injection of 100-200 mg/kg in guinea pigs [33].

Anti-Oxidant Effects

Polysaccharides (BCPS-1), isolated from *Bupleurum chinense* DC., has a backbone of (1→5)-linked Ara, (1→4)-linked Gal and (1→3)-linked Gal residues with occasionally branches at O-6. The branches composed of (1→4)-linked Glc, and terminated with Gal residues. *In vitro* antioxidant activity showed that BCPS-1 had a significant anti-oxidant effect in a concentration-dependent manner [68].

Cardiovascular Effects

Saikosaponins and ethanol extract had a negative inotropic effect on *in vitro* frog heart, which was not blocked by atropine. Blood pressure was slightly lowered in these test animals [33]. Different administrations were trialled. Intravenous injection of ethanol extract and Saikosaponins from *Buplerum chinense* DC. (5 ml/kg) produced no effect on blood pressure, breath or heart in rats nor in mice with subcutaneous injection (0.2 ml/kg) [33]. Further impact on cardiovascular diseases was observed in one study of herbal formula Saiko-ka-ryukotsu-borei-to (Chai Hu jia Long Gu Mu Li Tang in Chinese) with chief herb Radix Bupleuri (Chai Hu). This herbal formula was fed to the diets of spontaneously hypertensive rats for six weeks. The treatment increased endothelial progenitor cells colony numbers significantly with a decrease in oxidative stress and without affecting blood pressure test subjects. However, it did not reduce the expression of nicotinamide adenine dinucleotide phosphate oxidase subunits in cardiovascular organs. Serum IL-6 level was significantly reduced [69].

Gastrointestinal Effects

Polysaccharide of *Bupleurum falcatum* L. was detected to significantly reduce gastric mucosal lesions induced by HCl-ethanol [70-72] and indomethacin [71, 73] in mice.

Saikosaponins inhibited secretions of gastric acid and increased the pH value when orally ingested in rats. This promoted the recovery of gastric ulcers induced by dilute acetic acid [33]. Saikosaponins also improved peristaltic action of small intestines in mice and rabbits *in vitro* as well as increased strength in the contraction of intestinum ileum induced by acetycholine. However, no increase of contractions caused by histamine was detected [33]. Overall, Radix Bupleuri (Chai Hu) exhibited a remarkable anti-ulcerative action on stress ulcers in mice [6, 18].

A herbal formula, Sho-saiko-to (Xiao Chai Hu Tang in Chinese), significantly elevated the intragastric pH in pylorus-ligated rats, but induced no change in the concentrations of tolbutamide dissolved in the gastric content. Findings from this study indicated that Sho-saiko-to had an inhibitory effect on the function of gastric emptying in rats [74].

Hepatoprotective Effects

Seven saponins and one sapogenol from the seeds of *Bupleurum falcatum* L. and thirteen oleanene saponins from the aerial parts of *Bupleurum rotundifolium* L. were compared for their hepatoprotective activity and hepatotoxicity. The 13,28-epoxy type saponins had hepatoprotectivity. Ursane type showed hepatotoxicity from middle concentration. The 11,13(18)-diene type saponins did not express hepatoprotective activity. The 28-acid type saponin which has a glucosyl carboxy group showed hepatoprotective action [75].

Saikosaponin a significantly inhibited in bovine cells at both mRNA and protein levels of bone morphogenetic proteins 4. Findings indicated that Saikosaponin a could down-regulate the expression of bone morphogenetic proteins 4 and inhibit hepatic stellate cell activation [76].

Saikosaiponins a and d in Radix Bupleurum (Chai Hu) were investigated to have promoted choleresis and inhibited hepatic impairment caused by typhoid vaccine, alcohol, carbon tetrachloride (CCl_4), mycotic rice and aminogalactose [33] as well as cytotoxicity [45] induced by D-glactosamine (GalN) [77]. Similarly, Saikosaponin a from *Bupleurum komarovianum Linez* [78] and Saikosaponin d have been found to inhibit hepatic impairment induced by CCl_4 in mice and rats respectively. Enhanced phagocytosis was observed [77]. Another study also showed that Saikosaponins a and d inhibited the proliferation and migration of hepatic stellate cells which impact the pathogenesis of liver inflammation and fibrogenesis [79]. Furthermore, *Bupleurum*-based formula Xiao Chai Hu Tang converted positive HBsAg to negative in chronic hepatitis patients [80]. Significant inhibition in the increase of glutamic-pyruvic transaminase and glutamic-oxalacetic transminase as well as reduction in hyaline degeneration and Glisson cells infiltration in rats was also detected [81]. Oral administration of Xiao Chai Hu Tang attenuated the hepatic fibrosis developed in mice after repeated doses of carbon tetrachloride [82].

When fried with vinegar or mixed with vinegar, *Bupleurum marginatum* Wall ex DC. significantly inhibited an increase of serum glutamic-pyruvic transaminase induced by CCl_4 and slightly lessened hepatic injury in mice [83].

Ethanolic extract of Saikosaponins in *Bupleurum kaoi*, a Bupleurum indigenous to Taiwan, was fractionated (R, F_1, F_2 and F_3) and studied. This *in vitro* study revealed that pre-treatment with *Bupleurum kaoi* extract or its fractions, except F_3, significantly protected primary hepatocytes against damage by CCl_4. The R and F_1 fractions had the highest Saikosaponins content and most effectively protected the liver from damage by CCl_4. Oral administration of *Bupleurum kaoi* (100 and 500 mg/kg), except F_3, three days before a single dose of CCl_4, significantly lowered the serum levels of hepatic enzyme markers. A pathological examination showed that lesions, including ballooning degeneration, necrosis, hepatitis and portal triaditis were partially healed by treatment with *Bupleurum kaoi* extract and fractions. Oxidative stress induced by CCl_4 led to lipid peroxidation (MDA) and changes in the levels of the antioxidant enzymes in the liver. All fractions, except F_3, markedly suppressed lipid peroxidation and reversed the activities of the antioxidant enzymes to the normal levels [84].

Anti-Tumour Effects

The extract of Radix Bupleurum (Chai Hu) activated adenylate cyclise, a regulatory enzyme, in ascites cancer cells in mice in a dose dependent manner [85].

Isolated fractions (including CH-1, CH-3 and CH-4) had a stabilising effect on the both high and low concentrations of adenylate cyclise in normal mice livers [86]. CH-5 and CH-7 inhibited adenylate cyclise activity in mouse livers in a dose-dependent manner within a concentration range [86]. Purified fraction of Radix Bupleurum (Chai Hu) activated anti-tumour effector cells in mice [87].

Both *in vivo* and *in vitro* studies demonstrated that acetone extract of *Bupleurum scorzonerifolium* inhibited proliferation and induce apoptosis in A549 human lung cancer cells. Acetone extract of *Bupleurum scorzonerifolium* had the ability to cause cell cycle arrest in G2/M phase, induce tubulin polymerization, and activate caspase-3 and -9 in A549 human lung cancer cells. Its induced apoptosis could be blocked by the broad caspase inhibitor z-VAD-fmk in majority [88].

Saikosaponin d significantly inhibited the increase of S_{180}, P_{638} cells and ascites cancer cells in mice and prolonged survival rate when administered orally or intraperitioneally [89].

Saponin-enriched fraction from *Bupleurum kaoi* in human non-small cell lung cancer A549 cells was investigated and findings showed that the activity of the Fas/Fas ligand apoptotic system might participate in the antiproliferative activity of saponin-enriched fraction in A549 cells [90].

Saikosaponins c significantly lowered levels of HBsAg in HBV-transfected human hepatoma cells culture medium. It also possessed activity in inhibiting HBV DNA replication; however, this inhibitory effect was not due to the cytotoxicity of Saikosaponin c or its effect on 2.2.15 cell proliferation [28].

Saikosaponin d exhibited cytotoxicity on cells but it failed to inhibit HBV multiplication. The cytotoxicity of Saikosaponin d against $HepG_2$ human hepatocellular carcinoma cells was due to the induction of apoptosis through the activation of caspases-3 and -7, which subsequently resulted in poly-ADP-ribose-polymerase cleavage. DNA fragmentation was noted after $HepG_2$ cells exposure to Saikosaponin d [28]. Saikosaponin d also had a cytotoxic effect on DU145 cells. Saikosaponin d inhibited DU145 cell proliferation in a concentration dependent manner. It arrested the cell cycle at G0/G1 phase via upregulation of p53 and p21 and induced apoptosis by modulating B cell lymphoma 2 family proteins, dissipation of the mitochondrial membrane potential, and release of cytochrome c into the cytosol and activation of caspase-3 [91].

When male Sprague-Dawley rats were orally administered normal chow pellets containing Xiao Chai Hu Tang and drank water containing N-nitrosomorpholine for eight weeks, higher concentration of Xiao Chai Hu Tang inhibited the development of γ-glutamyl transpeptidase-positive and glutathione-S-transferase-positive lesions, but was less effective than the lower concentration administration. Administration of the lower dose caused a significant increase in the proportion of helper T lymphocytes and a significant decrease in the labelling index of pre-neoplastic lesions. These findings indicated that Xiao Chai Hu Tang inhibited the development of hepatic foci [92].

One study investigated whether Radix Bupleuri (Chai Hu) extract enhanced 5-fluorouracil-induced cytotoxicity in $HepG_2$ hepatoma cells, while protecting normal blood lymphocytes. Radix Bupleurum (Chai Hu) increased the micronuclei frequency and DNA damage, resulting from 5-fluorouracil treatment. However, when human lymphocytes were co-treated with Radix Bupleurum (Chai Hu) and 5-fluorouracil, the frequency of 5-fluorouracil-induced micronuclei decreased. When cells were treated with 20 mu M 5-fluorouracil and 200 mu g/ml Radix Bupleurum (Chai Hu) simultaneously, Bax protein increased in $HepG_2$ cells at 24 hour; however, p21 and p53 proteins were up-regulated in normal human lymphocytes. Co-treatment with 200 mu g/ml Radix Bupleurum (Chai Hu) and 20 mu M 5-fluorouracil resulted in cell arrest at the late G_1/early S phase in $HepG_2$ cells and normal lymphocytes. In addition, Radix Bupleurum (Chai Hu) and 5-fluorouracil treatment increased mitochondria membrane potential collapse only in $HepG_2$ cells, while it was not changed in lymphocytes [93].

Metabolic Effects

Saikosaponins suppressed lipodieresis induced by adrenalin and adrenocorticotropic hormone, and inhibited insulin to reduce formation of fats [33]. They also decreased blood levels of cholesterol, triglycerates, lipolipids and triglycerides, and accelerate the faecal excretion of 14C-cholestrol and its metabolites in hyperlipidaemic rats [4, 6]. Increased blood glucose promoted the utilization ration of glucose in the biosynthesis of total lipids and cholesterol as well as enhanced incorporation of protein in rats with mixture of Saikosaponins a, c and d [33]. All test subjects were administered intramuscularly [4, 6, 33]. These Saikosaponins suppressed activity of Na^+, K^+ -ATP enyzmes and caused metabolic changes resulting in increased ACTH, aldehyde ketone and vassopressin secretion and inhibited activity of $_C$AMP phosphodiesterase [94].

α-Spinasterol and Bupleurol also markedly reduced plasma cholesterol level of animals on a high cholesterol diet [4, 6, 10].

Haemolytic Effects

Saikosaponins inhibited leucine aminopetidase (LAP), a cellular enzyme implicated in a number of pathological disorders [77]. Decocted Radix Bupleurum (Chai Hu) and Saikosaponins from *Bupleurum falcatum* L. produced strong haemolytic actions in several studies [89, 95]. However, in one recent study, contrary results were yielded on haemolytic activities of

Bupleurum chinense DC. saponins and its adjuvant potentials on the immune responses of ICR mice against ovalbumin. *Bupleurum chinense* DC. saponins showed only a slightly haemolytic effect, with its haemolytic percents being 3.32% and 1.19% at the concentrations of 500 and 250 μg/ml, respectively. *Bupleurum chinense* DC. saponins significantly enhanced concanavalin A-, lipopolysaccharide- and ovalbumin-stimulated splenocyte proliferation as well as ovalbumin-specific IgG, IgG_1 and IgG_{2b} antibody levels in serum. Overall results suggested that *Bupleurum chinense* DC. saponins could be safely used as adjuvant with low or non-haemolytic effect [96].

Anti-Radiative Effects

Bupleurum polysaccharides showed an anti-radiative effect in mice [97]. Crude polysaccharides from the anti-UVB *Buplerum scorzonerifolium* cell clone inhibited UVB-induced photodamage (HaCaT cell death) without inducing any cytotoxic effect using a human skin keratinocyte cell line. Decreased reactive oxygen species and lipid peroxidation and increased superoxide dismutase activity indicated that crude polysaccharides acted as a free radical scavenger. Furthermore, crude polysaccharides had a strong protective ability against UVB-induced DNA damage. The portion of crude polysaccharides from the anti-UVB *Bupleurum scorzonerifolium* cell clone was more than 2.5-fold higher than crude polysaccharides from normal *Bupleurum scorzonerifolium* callus. The protective mechanisms of crude polysaccharides from the anti-UVB *Bupleurum scorzonerifolium* cell occur by the inhibition of UVB-induced reactive oxygen species production, lipid peroxidation and DNA damage [98].

Anti-Depressive Effects

Butanol and aqueous fractions obtained from the 60% ethanol extract of *Bupleurum chinense* DC. were studied on lipid peroxidation in chronic unpredictable mild stress model of depression in rats, and lymphocyte proliferation in mice. The effects of the serum of mice treated with butanol fraction or aqueous fraction on the lymphocyte proliferation *in vitro* was determined by MTT (3-(4,5-dimethylthiazol-2-yl)-2,5-diphenyltetrazolium bromide) tetrazolium reduction assay (a cell viability assay). Findings demonstrated that aqueous and fraction or butanol fraction enhanced activities of superoxide dismutase, glutathione peroxidase and catalase, significantly reduced the malondialdehyde content in serum in rats with chronic unpredictable mild stress. They also concentration-dependently increased concanavalin A-induced proliferation of spleen lymphocytes, and 20% concentration of serum had a better effect. The possible mechanism of butanol and aqueous fractions for anti-depressive action may be involved in anti-oxidation and the drug serum could reinforce immune function, hence combination with antidepressant may improve the anti-depressive effect [99]. Xiao Yao San, a famous Chinese herbal formula composing of Radix Bupleuri (Chai Hu) as a chief herb, has been widely used for treating mental disorders. Behaviour and biochemical analyses indicated it had obvious anti-depressive activity. However, there is no report on the effects of Xiao Yao San using a metabolomics approach [100].

Total Saikosaponins from *Bupleurum yinchowense* exhibited an effect on acute stress and chronic unpredictable mild stress models in an *in vivo* experiment. The PC12 cells were treated with corticosterone in the absence or presence of different concentrations of total Saikosaponins. Findings showed that pre-treatment of PC12 cells with total Saikosaponins partly reversed corticosterone-induced neurotoxicity in a dose dependent manner. Total Saikosaponins also reversed the increase of dead cells in the Hoechst 33342 stain, the accumulation in lactate dehydrogenase leakage and the number of TUNEL positive cells induced by corticosterone to PC12 cells. Moreover, the cytoprotection of total Saikosaponins was proven to be associated with the homeostasis of intracellular Ca^{2+}, the stabilization of endoplasmic reticulum (ER) stress via the down-regulation of glucose-regulated protein 78, DNA damage inducible proteins 153, X-box DNA-binding protein-1, and the restoration of mitochondrial function, which included mitochondrial permeability transition pore, mitochondrial membrane potential and caspase-3 activity. Total Saikosaponins markedly ameliorated up-regulation of Bax and down-regulation of Bcl-2 in corticosterone-induced PC12 cells. The results depicted that the antidepressant-like effect of total Saikosaponins *in vivo* may be associated with the cytoprotection of neurons, and the neuroprotective mechanisms were correlated with inhibiting the ER stress and the mitochondrial apoptotic pathways [101].

One study investigated the impact of *Bupleurum falcatum* L. extract on repeated restraint stress-induced behavioural responses using the forced swimming test and elevated plus maze test. Findings showed that repeated restraint stress in rodents produced increases in depression and anxiety-like behaviours and altered the expression of corticotrophin-releasing factor in the hypothalamus. Hypothalamic-pituitary-adrenal axis activation in response to repeated restraint stress was confirmed based on serum corticosterone levels and corticotrophin-releasing factor expression in the hypothalamus. Animals that were pre-treated with *Bupleurum falcatum* L. extract significantly reduced immobility in the forced swimming test and increased open-arm exploration in the elevated plus maze test in comparison with controls. *Bupleurum falcatum* L. also blocked the increase in tyroxine hydroxylase expression in the locus coeruleus of treated rats that experienced restraint stress [102].

Anti-Osteoclast Effects

Five new Saikosaponins that include *Saikosaponin* w, 21β-hydroxysaikosaponin b_2, 6″-O-acetylsaikosaponin e, 6″-O-acetylsaikosaponin b_1, and 6″-O-acetylsaikosaponin b_3, were isolated from the roots of *Bupleurum chinense* DC [103]. Osteoclast-inhibiting activity of some of the isolated compounds was evaluated *in vitro*, with five new showing significant activity by inhibitory rates ranging from 48.3% to 56.1% at the concentration of 10 μM and with significant differences among groups observed [103].

Anti-Nephritis Effects

Effects of Saikosaponins a, c, and d from *Bupleurum scorzonerifolium* and *Bupleurum falcatum* L. were compared. Five treatments of Saikosaponin a, Saikosaponin c, or Saikosaponin d were administered to nephritic mice. Saikosaponin c almost completely prevented the development of nephritis, although immune-complex deposition was not affected. Saikosaponin d from *Bupleurum falcatum* L. had a significant but lesser effect. Saikosaponin a from *Bupleurum falcatum* L. did not show any effect [104].

Xiao Chai Hu Tang could protect type-1 diabetic mice against diabetic nephropathy, using streptozotocin (STZ)-induced diabetic mice and high-glucose (HG)-exposed rat mesangial cell (RMC) as models. Renal functions and renal hypertrophy significantly improved in the STZ-diabetic mice, while serum glucose was only moderately reduced compared to vehicle treatment. Treatment with Xiao Chai Hu Tang in the STZ-diabetic mice and HG-exposed RMC resulted in a decrease in expression levels of transforming growth factor beta 1 (TGF-β_1), fibronectin, and collagen IV, with concomitant increase in bone morphogenetic protein-7 expression. Data indicated that Xiao Chai Hu

Tang could scavenge free radicals and inhibit high-glucose-induced reactive oxidative stress in rat mesangial cells [105]. The outcome of this study suggested that treatment with Xiao Chai Hu Tang could improve renal function during the development of diabetic nephropathy.

Anti-Allergic Effects

Saikosaponin d was investigated on the effect of allergic reactions caused by β-conglycinin, using a rat basophilic leukemia-2H3 cell line. There were multiple signalling pathways contributing to the development of β-conglycinin-mediated rat basophilic leukemia-2H3 cell activation. The intracellular calcium mobilisation and tyrosine phosphorylation were early events, which in turn elicited reactive oxygen species production, gene activation of Cdc42 and c-Fos, and ultimately led to β-hexosaminidase release. Saikosaponin d inhibited rat basophilic leukemia-2H3 cell degranulation by suppressing these critical incidents in the signal transduction pathway [106].

Anti-Thrombotic & Anti-Platelets Aggregation Effects

Saikosaponins from *Bupleurum rigidum* significantly inhibited human platelets aggregation induced by Adenosine diphosphate and dose-dependently suppressed platelet thromboxane formation from arachidonic acid [107]. When administered intraperitoneally, Xiao Chai Hu Tang (200 mg/kg) inhibited capillary permeability and released inhibition of adrenocorticotropic hormone (ACTH) secretion induced by corticosterone [29]. With the dosage of 1.1 g/kg (ten times more than human dosage), its anti-inflammatory effect is equivalent to that of 1 mg/kg of hydroprednisone [108]. This formula had an inhibitory effect on $FeCl_3$-induced thrombus formation through anti-platelet activity *in vitro*, and significantly inhibited various agonist-induced platelet aggregations, including serotonin secretion and thromboxane B_2 formation [109]. Xiao Chai Hu Tang also prolonged the occlusion time of thrombus formation when applied to a $FeCl_3$-induced thrombus formation model, and suppressed collagen-induced platelet aggregation *ex vivo* in a concentration-dependent manner. However, it did not affect coagulation [109].

Chloroformic crude extract of roots of *Bupleurum fruticosum* L. (Umbelliferae) lowered intracellular calcium concentration. Vasorelaxing effect on aortic rings endothelium-deprived and pre-contracted by norepinephrine (NE) was yielded with concentration-dependent Bupleurum extract. The pharmacological effect was not produced through the stimulation of cyclooxygenase, adenyl cyclase, or guanylyl cyclase, since selective inhibitors did not prevent the extract-induced responses. It was noted aortic rings with the chloroformic extract produced a depression of the concentration-contractile response curve to NE, more evident in Ca^{2+}-free Tyrode solution, suggesting an action on the intracellular mobilization of Ca^{2+} ions. Moreover, the vasodilator action of *Bupleurum fruticosum* L. extract was resistant to the pre-treatment with nifedipine and to the pre-treatment with cyclopiazonic acid (blocker of Ca^{2+}/ATPase). Finally, the chloroformic extract of *Bupleurum fruticosum* L. reduced the contraction obtained by caffeine, an opener of ryanodine-sensitive receptors [110].

Pharmacokinetics

Administration and Absorption

Saponins in Radix Bupleuri (Chai Hu) were found hard to absorb orally. It is found some are rendered inactive in the digestive tract. Similarly, oral administration of saponins only gained one tenth of the anti-inflammatory effects to that of intramuscular injection of the same dosage [33]. However, intramuscular administration of Radix Bupleuri (Chai Hu) could cause asthma [111, 112], urticaria [113] and allergic shock [114, 115].

A paired herb Chai Hu-Shao Yao that has been widely used for anti-inflammatory purpose was studied *in vivo* for its absorption rate using a four-site perfused rat intestinal model. Saikosaponin a, Saikosaponin d and paeoniflorin are identified as the main components in the pair. All of the three main components displayed very low permeabilities, which implied their poor absorption in the rat intestines. The absorption levels of Saikosaponin a and Saikosaponin d were similar in intestines and higher in ileum than those in other intestinal regions in the decreasing order: colon, jejunum and duodenum. Evidence showed that Saikosaponin a and Saikosaponin d could promote the absorption of paeoniflorin [116].

Excretion

Bupleuri clearance is slow and mainly through faecal excretion. Saikosaponins a and d are excreted through faeces 50% on the 2nd day and 85% on the 7th day. Some are excreted through the urinary tract [6].

Drugs Metabolism

After the Sprague-Dawley rats were administered for seven days, the original and vinegar-baked Radix Bupleuri (Chai Hu) demonstrated different effects on the CYP2C9 and CYP2C19. The original Radix Bupleuri (Chai Hu) decreased plasma concentration of omeprazole, but treatment of vinegar-baked type with normal dose did not change the pharmacokinetics of omeprazole. The pharmacokinetics of tolbutamide in all vinegar-baked Radix Bupleuri (Chai Hu)-treated rats showed no statistically significant difference from that of controlled rats; however, treatment of the original type decreased tolbutamide. The pharmacokinetics of caffeine displayed no significant difference in rats treated by either the original or vinegar-baked type [117].

Toxicology

Minimal lethal dose of 10% Bupleurum ethanol extract was 1.1 ml/10g in mice [33]. and 100 mg/kg in guinea pigs [6]. Median lethal dose (LD_{50}) varies depending on the type of animal test subjects and the methods of administration.

LD_{50} value of Saikosaponin was 4.7 g/kg orally [33], 1.9 g/kg subcutaneously and 70 mg/kg intravenously in mice as well as 58.3 mg/kg in guinea pigs and 479 mg/kg in mice intraperitoneally [4]. LD_{50} value of volatile oil of *Bupleurum chinense* DC. was 1.19 ± 0.12 g/kg in mice when administered intraperitoneally [21].

LD_{50} of *Radix Bupleuri longiradiatum* was 500 mg/kg in mice when orally consumed in granule. Toxicity of Radix Bupleuri (Chai Hu) injection is extremely low [4].

LD_{50} of Bupleururotoxin at 3.03 mg/kg and acetyl-bupleuruotxin at 3.13 mg/kg [4]. *Bupleurum longiradiatum* Turcz. (Da Ye Chai Hu) is highly toxic and not to be used as alternative for Radix Bupleuri (Chai Hu).

One study was conducted in Taiwan to investigate the association between the use of Chinese herbal products containing Radix Bupleuri (Chai Hu) and the risk of hospitalisation related to liver injury among patients infected by hepatitis B virus (HBV). A total of 1,080 cases were included for analysis after screening 639,779 patients with diagnoses related to HBV infection. The risks from prescribing the Xiao Chai Hu Tang and Long Dan Xie Gan Tang were significantly high and dose-response relationships were found. Findings revealed that prescribing Xiao Chai Hu Tang, Long Dan Xie Gan Tang or Chinese herbal products containing more than nineteen grams of Radix Bupleuri (Chai Hu) in HBV-infected patients might increase their risks of liver injury [118].

Clinical Side Effects

Increased sedative effects with increased bowel movements, flatulence and sedation were noted [119]. About 30% of patients experienced symptoms of mild lassitude, sedation and drowsiness after a small dose of 0.6 g of the herb in powder form consumed orally [119]. Sedative effects did not affect daily activities in the patients tested. Larger doses caused deep sedation in 80% of the subjects tested and 17% experienced poor sleep [120].

Gastrointestinal irritation, abdominal distension, loss of appetite, constipation and facial and extreme oedema were observed in clinical trials when large doses of Radix Bupleuri (Chai Hu) of 2 g/d were consumed [121].

Pneumonitis was associated with Xiao Chai Hu Tang during the treatment of chronic active hepatitis in Japan [122].

Intramuscular administration of Radix Bupleuri (Chai Hu) could cause allergic effects such as asthma [111, 112], urticaria [113] and allergic shock (3 cases) [114, 115].

Interactions

Herb to herb adverse interaction was noted when mixed injection of Radix Bupleuri (Chai Hu) and Radix Isatidis (Ban Lan Gen) administered intramuscularly. Allergic shock has been reported one case [123].

Herb to drug adverse reaction is rendered when mixed injection of Radix Bupleuri (Chai Hu) with Antondine [6] or Gentamicin [124] when administered intramuscularly. Allergic shocks were reported. Combination of IFN-α and Xiao Chai Hu Tang for chronic active hepatitis caused pneumonitis [122]. Decreased blood concentrations was noted when taken with Xiao Chai Hu Tang with prednisolone [125].

Dosages

Dosages should be restricted to amount recommended in the Pharmacopoeia of People's Republic of China [3]. Large doses should be avoided and not intended for long-term use. Recommended dose is within 9-12 g per prescription [1].

Quality Control

Roots of *Bupleurum chinense* DC. and *Bupleurum scorzonerifolium* are indigenous Chinese Materia Medica in China [1, 5, 9]. Some other species such as the roots of *Bupleurum falcatum* L., *Bupleurum bicaule* and *Bupleurum marginatum var. stenophyllum* which have similar actions to Chai Hu can also occasionally be found in local raw herb markets. Good quality bupleurum has a long and thick root, and a thin cortex, with few rootlets [1, 6]. Total ash is not more than 8.0% and the extractives are not less than 11.0% using ethanol as solvent following the hot extraction method [3].

Precautions and Guidelines for Safe Prescription

Chinese medicine practitioners should exercise extreme caution when prescribing Radix Bupleuri (Chai Hu) with children and not to prescribe Radix Bupleuri (Chai Hu) during pregnancy and lactation in women. Large doses in both adults and children prescription and long term use should best be avoided [3]. Chinese medicine practitioners have to check quality control of Radix Bupleuri (Chai Hu) during processing with suppliers, and ensure clear distinction identification between *Bupleuri longiradiatum* Turcz. (De Ye Chai Hu) and Radix Bupleuri (Chai Hu) to avoid toxic constituents. There is a need to avoid prescribing Radix Bupleuri (Chai Hu) for patients who are prone to allergic reactions. Practitioners also have to differentiate syndromes to avoid contraindications in herbal prescription especially Radix Bupleuri (Chai Hu) with Radix Isatidis (Ban Lan Gen), Antondine, Gentamincin or interferon treatment. Patients should be advised not to self prescribe Radix Bupleuri (Chai Hu). Importantly, Chinese medicine practitioners should advise their patients' Western medicine practitioner, should they be administering Radix Bupleuri (Chai Hu). Finally, all Chinese medicine practitioners should be formally trained in understanding the properties, actions, indications, contraindications, interactions, dosage and usage of this herb before prescribing it.

Current Regulations

Both raw herb and the extract of Radix Bupleuri (Chai Hu) are currently not scheduled in Australia [126], European Union [127], or People's Republic of China [128]. In Hong Kong, Radix Bupleuri (Chai Hu) is a Schedule 2 herb and is available in retail, wholesale and can only be dispensed by a licensed person [129].

References

[1] Bensky, D; Gamble, A. Chinese herbal medicine: Materia medica. revised ed. Seattle: Eastland Press, 1993.
[2] Li, JS; Jia, MR. Zhongyao jiandingxue [Identification of Chinese herbal medicine]. Shanghai: Shanghai Scientific and Technical Publishers, 1996.
[3] The Pharmacopoeia Commission of People's Republic of China, editor. Pharmacopoeia of the People's Republic of China (English edition). Beijing: Chemical Industry Press, 2000.
[4] Zhu, YP. Chinese materia medica: Chemistry, pharmacology and applications. Singapore: Harwood Academic Publishers, 1998.
[5] Lei, ZQ; Chen, SY; Gao, XM; Guo, ZQ; editors. Zhongyaoxue [Chinese Materia Medica]. Shanghai: Shanghai Scientific and Technical Publishers, 1995.

[6] State Administration of Traditional Chinese Medicine "Chinese Materia Medica" Committee, editor. Zhonghua bencao [Chinese materia medica]. Shanghai: Shanghai Scientific and Technical Publishers, 1998.

[7] Bermejo, Benito, P; Abad, Martinez, MJ; Silvan, Sen, AM; Sanz, Gomez, A; Fernandez, Matellano, L; Sanchez, Contreras, S; et al. In vivo and in vitro antiinflammatory activity of saikosaponins. *Life Sci.*, 1998, 63(13), 1147-56.

[8] Estevez-Braun, A; Estevez-Reyes, R; Moujie, LM; Ravelo, AG; Gonzalez, AG. Antibiotic activity and absolute configuration of 8s-heptadeza-2(z),9(z)-diene-4,6-diyne-1,8-diol from bupleurum salicifolium. *J Nat Prod.*, 1994, 57(8), 1178-82.

[9] Jiangsu, Xin, Yi, Xue, Yuan; editor. Zhongyao dacidian [Grand dictionary of Chinese herbal medicine]. Shanghai: Shanghai Scientific and Technical Publishers, 1986.

[10] Chang, WC; Hsu, FL. Inhibition of platelet activation and endothelial cell injury by flavan-3-ol and saikosaponin compounds. *Prostaglandins Leukot Essent Fatty Acids.*, 1991, 44, 51-6.

[11] Guo, JX; Pan, SL; Li, Y; Hong, XK; Wang, ZH. Zhongguo Chaihushu 19 zhong zhiwu huifayou huaxue chengfen de yanjiu [Study on the chemical constituents of 19 volatile oils from Bupleurum in China]. *ACTA Academiae Medicinae Shanghai.*, 1990, 17(4), 278-82.

[12] Yan, XJ; Milne, GWA; Zhou, JJ; Xie, GR. Traditional Chinese medicines: Molecular structures, natural sources, and applications. Aldershot, Great Britain: Ashgate, 1999.

[13] Geng, JX; Chen, SR. Chai Hu duotang de fenli he jianding [Isolation and identification of polysaccharides from radix Bupleuri]. *Zhongguo Zhong Yao Za Zhi [China Journal of Chinese Materia Medica].*, 1989, 14(1), 37-40, 63.

[14] Luo, SQ; Jin, HF. Bei Chai Hu jingye de huaxue chengfen yanjiu [Study on chemical constituents from the rhizoma of Bupleurum chinense DC.]. *Zhong Yao Tong Bao.*, 1988, 13(1), 36-8.

[15] Gao, G; Guo, YZ. Chai Hu shu 12 zhong Chai Hu de zhiliang pingjia yanjiu [Evaluation of 12 species of Bupleurum]. *Zhong Cao Yao.*, 1988, 19(10), 11-4.

[16] Jia, Q; Zhang, RY. Chai Hu shu zhi wuzhong zaodai huaxue yanjiu jinzhan [Study on five saikosaponins from Radix Bupleuri]. *Aclia Pharmaceutica Sinica.*, 1989, 24(12), 961-71.

[17] Dong, YY; Luo, SQ; Pan, SL. Chai Hu zhuyao zaodai chengfen de gaoxiao yexiang sepu ceding [Determination of saikosaponins in radix

Bupleuri using HPLC]. *China Journal of Chinese Materia Medica.*, 1989, 14(11), 678-81, 703-4.

[18] Dong, ZL; Yu, SF. Modern study and application of materia medica. Hong Kong: China Ocean Press, 1990.

[19] Qin, X; Dai, Y; Liu, NQ; Li, Z; Liu, X; Hu, J; et al. Metabolic fingerprinting by 1HNMR for discrimination of the two species used as Radix Bupleuri. *Planta Med.*, 2012, 78(9), 926-33. Epub, 2012/04/28.

[20] Liang, Z; Oh, K; Wang, Y; Yi, T; Chen, H; Zhao, Z. Cell type-specific qualitative and quantitative analysis of saikosaponins in three Bupleurum species using laser microdissection and liquid chromatography-quadrupole/time of flight-mass spectrometry. *J Pharm Biomed Anal.*, 2014, 97, 157-65.

[21] Zhou, ZC; Zhou, QL; Wang, BX. Bei Chai Hu he Da Ye Chai Hu yaoli zuoyong de bijiao [Pharmacological comparison between Bupleurum chinense DC. and B. longeradiatum Turcz.]. *Yao Xue Tong Bao.*, 1979, 14(6), 252-4.

[22] Martin, S; Padilla, E; Ocete, MA; Galvez, J; Jimenez, J; Zarzuelo, A. Anti-inflammatory activity of the essential oil of Bupleurum fruticescens. *Planta Med.*, 1993, 59, 533-6.

[23] Lorente, I; Ocete, MA; Zarzuelo, A; Cabo, MM; Jimenez, J. Bioactivity of the essential oil of bupleurum fruticosum. *J Nat Prod.*, 1989, 52(2), 267-72.

[24] Just, MJ; Recio, MC; Giner, RM; Cuellar, MJ; Manez, S; Bilia, j-LR; et al. Anti-inflammatory activity of unusual lupane saponins from bupleurum fruticescens. *Planta Med.*, 1998, 64, 404-7.

[25] Xie, Y; Lu, W; Cao, S; Jiang, X; Yin, M; Tang, W. Preparation of bupleurum nasal spray and evaluation on its safety and efficacy. *Chem Pharm Bull (Tokyo).*, 2006, 54(1), 48-53. Epub, 2006/01/06.

[26] Chu, XH; Hou, XD. Chai Hu ji Gui Zhi zhiliao duofaxing jiyan de shiyan yanjiu [Experimental study on polymyositis by Radix Bupleuri and Ramulus Cinnamomi]. *Chinese Journal of Integrated Traditional and Western Medicine.*, 1998, 18(6), 356-8.

[27] Li, X-Q; He, Z-G; Bi, K-S; Song, Z-H; Liang, X. Essential oil analyses of the root oils of 10 Bupleurum species from China. *J Essent Oil Res.*, 2007, 19(3), 234-8.

[28] Phytotherapy; Saikosaponins from Bupleurum exhibit antiviral and anticancer, properties. *Hepatitis Weekly.*, 2003 Dec 1, 24.

[29] Wu, ZF; Xiong, CM; Zhang, JB. Chai Hu zhusheye jiere kangyan zuoyong de chubu yanjiu [Study on antipyretic and anti-inflammatory

effects of Bupleurum injection]. *Chinese Journal of Pharmaceutical Analysis.*, 1983, 3(5), 293-6.

[30] Lu, C-N; Yuan, Z-G; Zhang, X-L; Yan, R; Zhao, Y-Q; Liao, M; et al. Saikosaponin a and its epimer saikosaponin d exhibit anti-inflammatory activity by suppressing activation of NF-κB signaling pathway. *Int Immunopharmacol.*, 2012, 14(1), 121-6.

[31] Ashour, ML; Wink, M. Genus Bupleurum: a review of its phytochemistry, pharmacology and modes of action. *J Pharm Pharmacol.*, 2011, 63(3), 305-21.

[32] Cao, F; Tang, A. Effects of Xiao-Chai-Hu decoction with different doses of Bupleurum on body temperature and content of IL-1β, IL-6, TNF-α in serum induced by LPS among fever rat models. *Modernization of Traditional Chinese Medicine and Materia Medica-World Science and Technology.*, 2014, 16(1), 58-62.

[33] Zhang, B. Chai Hu shu zhiwu de yaoli zuoyong yanjiu gaikuang [Study on pharmacology of Bupleurum species]. *Jilin Zhong Yi Yao.*, 1983(1), 39-41.

[34] Di, HY; Zhang, YY; Chen, DF. Isolation of an anti-complementary polysaccharide from the root of Bupleurum chinense and identification of its targets in complement activation cascade. *Chin J Nat Med.*, 2013, 11(2), 177-84. Epub, 2013/06/22.

[35] Cheng, X-Q; Li, H; Yue, X-L; Xie, J-Y; Zhang, Y-Y; Di, H-Y; et al. Macrophage immunomodulatory activity of the polysaccharides from the roots of Bupleurum smithii var. parvifolium. *J Ethnopharmacol.*, 2010, 130(2), 363-8.

[36] Jiang, Y-W; Li, H; Zhang, Y-Y; Li, W; Jiang, Y-F; Ou, Y-Y; et al. Beneficial effect of Bupleurum polysaccharides on autoimmune-prone MRL-lpr mice. *Clin Dev Immunol.*, 2012, 842928.

[37] Zhang, XQ; Chen, HS. Chai Hu duotang de mianyi yaoli zuoyong [Immunology of Bupleurum polysaccharides]. *Chin J Pharmacol Toxicol.*, 1989, 3(1), 30-3.

[38] Wu, J; Zhang, Y-Y; Guo, L; Li, H; Chen, D-F. Bupleurum polysaccharides attenuates lipopolysaccharide-induced inflammation via modulating toll-like receptor 4 signaling: e78051. *PLoS One.*, 2013, 8(10).

[39] Tong, H; Tian, D; Li, T; Wang, B; Jiang, G; Sun, X. Inhibition of inflammatory injure by polysaccharides from Bupleurum chinense through antagonizing P-selectin. *Carbohydrate Polymers.*, 2014, 105(0), 20-5.

[40] Zuo, ZP; Wang, ZB; Gao, Y; Guo, YD; Wang, BS; Su, B; et al. Chai Hu zhusheye tiwai yizhi PGE_2 shifang de shengwu huoxing cedingfa [Bioactivity assay of bupleurum injection for inhibiting PGE2 release in vitro]. *China Journal of Chinese Materia Medica.*, 2013, 38(22), 3957-60. Epub, 2014/02/25.

[41] Wu, J; Zhang, YY; Guo, L; Li, H; Chen, DF. Bupleurum polysaccharides attenuates lipopolysaccharide-induced inflammation via modulating Toll-like receptor 4 signaling. *PLoS One.*, 2013, 8(10), e78051. Epub, 2013/10/30.

[42] Kawakita, T; Nakai, S; Kumazawa, W; Miura, O; Yumioka, E; Nomoto, K. Induction of interferon after administration of a traditional Chinese medicine, xiao-chai-hu-tang (shosaiko-to). *Int J Immunopharmacol.*, 1990, 5(12).

[43] Cheng, PW; Ng, LT; Lin, CC. Xiao chai hu tang inhibits CVB1 virus infection of CCFS-1 cells through the induction of Type I interferon expression. *Int Immunopharmacol.*, 2006, 6(6), 1003-12.

[44] Piras, G; Makino, M; Baba, M. Sho-Saiko-To, a traditional kampo medicine, ehnaces teh anti-HIV-1 activity of lamuvudine (3TC) in vitro. *Microbiol Immunology.*, 1997, 41(10), 835-9.

[45] Ashour, ML; El-Readi, MZ; Hamoud, R; Eid, SY; El, Ahmady, SH; Nibret, E; et al. Anti-infective and cytotoxic properties of Bupleurum marginatum. *Chinese Medicine.*, 2014, 9, 4.

[46] Bermejo, P; Abad, MJ; Diaz, AM; Fernandez, L; De, Santos, J; Sanchez, S; et al. Antiviral activity of seven iridoids, three saikosaponins and one phenylpropanoid glycoside extracted from Bupleurum rigidum and Scrophularia scorodonia. *Planta Med.*, 2002, 68(2), 106-10. Epub, 2002/02/23.

[47] Ushio, Y; Oda, Y; Abe, H. Effect of saikosaponin on the immune responses in mice. *Int J Immunopharmacol.*, 1991, 13(5), 501-8.

[48] Kato, M; Pu, M-Y; Isobe, K-I; Iwamoto, T; Nagase, F; Lwin, T; et al. Characterization of the immunoregulatory action of saikosaponin-d. *Cell Immunol.*, 1994, 159, 15-25.

[49] Chow, LW; Loo, WT; Sham, JS. Effects of a herbal compound containing bupleurum on human lymphocytes. *Hong Kong Med J.*, 2001, 7(4), 408-13.

[50] Guo, Y; Matsumoto, T; Kikuchi, Y; Ikejima, T; Wang, B; Yamada, H. Effects of a pectic polysaccharide from a medicinal herb, the roots of Bupleurum falcatum L. on interleukin 6 production of murine B cells and B cell lines. *Immunopharmacology.*, 2000, 49(3), 307-16.

[51] Wang, Z; Li, H; Xu, H; Yue, X-L; Cheng, X-Q; Hou, W-J; et al. Beneficial effect of Bupleurum polysaccharides on autoimmune disease induced by Campylobacter jejuni in BALB/c mice. *J Ethnopharmacol.*, 2009, 124(3), 481-7.

[52] Jung, DW; Shibuya, M; Ebizuka, Y; Yoshimatsu, K; Shimomura, K; Sung, CK. ELISA for the determination of saikosaponin a, an active component of Bupleuri Radix. *Chem Pharm Bull (Tokyo).*, 1998, 46(7), 1140-3.

[53] Izumi, S; Ohno, N; Kawakita, T; Nomoto, K; Yadomae, T. Wide range of molecular weight distribution of mitogenic substance(s) in the hot water extract of a Chinese herbal medicine, Bupleurum chinense. *Biol Pharm Bull.*, 1997, 20(7), 759-64.

[54] Oka, H; Ohno, N; Iwanaga, S; Izumi, S; Kawakita, T; Nomoto, K; et al. Characterization of mitogenic substances in the hot water extracts of bupleuri radix. *Biol Pharm Bull.*, 1995, 18(5), 757-65.

[55] Kim, H; Kim, SH; Yun, KW. Antioxidant activity and total phenolic contents of three Bupleurum taxa. *Nat Prod Commun.*, 2014, 9(4), 523-4. Epub, 2014/05/30.

[56] Wu, DJ. Chai Hu zhusheye zhiliao danbaobingdu jiaomoyan linchuang guancha [Clinical observation of effects of Bupleurum injection on herpes simplex keratitis]. *Zhong Cao Yao Tong Xun.*, 1978(12), 29.

[57] Gan, HS; Chen, SW. Bei Chai Hu gen yu jingye de zhiliang bijiao [Comparison between the root and rhizoma of Bupleurum chinense DC.]. *Zhongyao Tong Bao.*, 1982(2), 7-8.

[58] Cao, S-L; Chen, E; Zhang, Q-Z; Jiang, X-G. A novel nasal delivery system of a Chinese traditional medicine, Radix Bupleuri, based on the concept of ion-activated in situ gel. *Arch Pharm Res.*, 2007, 30(8), 1014-9.

[59] Chen, E; Chen, J; Cao, S-L; Zhang, Q-Z; Jiang, X-G. Preparation of nasal temperature-sensitive in situ gel of Radix Bupleuri and evaluation of the febrile response mechanism. *Drug Dev Ind Pharm.*, 2010, 36(4), 490-6.

[60] Chen, J-X; Ji, B; Lu, Z-L; Hu, L-S. Effects of Chai Hu (Radix Burpleuri) containing formulation on plasma β-endorphin, epinephrine and dopamine in patients. *Am J Chin Med.*, 2005, 33(05), 737-45.

[61] Lee, B; Shim, I; Lee, H; Hahm, D-H. Effect of Bupleurum falcatum on the stress-induced impairment of spatial working memory in rats. *Biol Pharm Bull.*, 2009, 32(8), 1392-8.

[62] Liu, Y; Wu, H; Ge, F. Chai Hu sanzhong cuiquwu kangjingjue zuoyong youxiao chengfen tantao [Chemical constituents analysis on anticonvulsive effect of three extracts from Radix Bupleuri]. *Zhong Yao Cai.*, 2002, 25(9), 635-7.

[63] Yu, YH; Xie, W; Bao, Y; Li, HM; Hu, SJ; Xing, JL. Saikosaponin a mediates the anticonvulsant properties in the HNC models of AE and SE by inhibiting NMDA receptor current and persistent sodium current. *PLoS One.*, 2012, 7(11), e50694. Epub, 2012/12/05.

[64] Sugaya, E; Ishige, A; Sekiguchi, K; Iizuka, S; Ito, K; Sugimoto, A; et al. Inhibitory effect of TJ-960 (SK) on pentylenetetrazol-induced EEG power spectrum changes. *Epilepsy Res.*, 1988, 2(1), 27-31.

[65] Wu, HM; Huang, CC; Li, LH; Tsai, JJ; Hsu, KS. The Chinese herbal medicine Chai-Hu-Long-Ku-Mu-Li-Tan (TW-001) exerts anticonvulsant effects against different experimental models of seizure in rats. *Jpn J Pharmacol.*, 2000, 82(3), 247-60.

[66] Xie, W; Yu, YH; Du, YP; Zhao, YY; Li, CZ; Yu, L; et al. Saikosaponin a enhances transient inactivating potassium current in rat hippocampal CA1 neurons. *Evid Based Complement Alternat Med.*, 2013, 2013, 413092. Epub, 2013/04/05.

[67] Xu, S-M; Zheng, K-J; He, J-Y. Chai Hu dui dianxian moxing dianhuodong de tiaozhi [Modulation with bupleurum root on brain electrical activities in epileptic model]. *Zhongguo Ying Yong Sheng Li Xue Za Zhi [Chinese Journal of Applied Physiology].*, 2002, 18(3), 294-6.

[68] Sun, L; Feng, K; Jiang, R; Chen, J; Zhao, Y; Ma, R; et al. Water-soluble polysaccharide from Bupleurum chinense DC: Isolation, structural features and antioxidant activity. *Carbohydr Polym.*, 2010, 79(1), 180-3.

[69] Iijima, H; Daikonya, A; Satoshi, T; Kanno, A; Magariyama, K; Yoshikawa, K; et al. Effects of the herbal medicine composition "Saiko-ka-ryukotsu-borei-To" on the function of endothelial progenitor cells in hypertensive rats. *Phytomedicine.*, 2013, 20(3-4), 196-201.

[70] Matsumoto, T; Moriguchi, R; Yamada, H. Role of polymorphonuclear leucocytes and oxygen-derived free radicals in the formation of gastric lesions induced by HCl/ethanol, and a possible mechanism of protection by anti-ulcer polysaccharide. *J Pharm Pharmacol.*, 1993, 45(6), 535-9.

[71] Shan, T; Yang, C. Chai Hu duotang chengfen zhi yanjiu (di 3 bao) [Study on constituents of bupleurum polysaccharide (3rd report)]. *Guo Wai Yi Xue - Zhong Yi Zhong Yao Fen Ce.*, 1991, 13(6), 39.

[72] Sun, XB. Chai Hu duotang dui shiyanxing weinianmo sunshang de baohu zuoyong [Protective effects on gastric mucosal injury caused by bupleurum polysaccharide]. *Jilin Zhong Yi Yao.*, 1991(6), 33-4.

[73] Sun, XB. Chaihu duotang chengfen zhi yanjiu (di 4 bao) [Study on constituents of bupleurum polysaccharide (4th report)]. *Guo Wai Yi Xue - Zhong Yi Zhong Yao Fen Ce.*, 1991, 13(6), 39.

[74] Nishimura, N; Naora, K; Hirano, H; Iwamoto, K. Effects of Sho-saiko-to (Xiao Chai Hu Tang), a Chinese traditional medicine, on the gastric function and absorption of tolbutamide in rats. *Yakugaku Zasshi.*, 2001, 121(2), 153-9.

[75] Nakahara, Y; Okawa, M; Kinjo, J; Nohara, T. Oleanene glycosides of the aerial parts and seeds of Bupleurum falcatum and the aerial parts of Bupleurum rotundifolium, and their evaluation as anti-hepatitis agents. *Chem Pharm Bull (Tokyo).*, 2011, 59(11), 1329-39. Epub, 2011/11/02.

[76] Wang, X; Wang, Q; Burczynski, FJ; Kong, W; Gong, Y. Saikosaponin a of Bupleurum chinense (Chaihu) elevates bone morphogenetic protein 4 (BMP-4) during hepatic stellate cell activation. *Phytomedicine.*, 2013, 20(14), 1330-5. Epub, 2013/08/24.

[77] Guinea, MC; Parellada, J; Lacaille-Dubois, MA; Wagner, H. Biologically active triterpene saponins from bupleurum fruticosum. *Planta Med.*, 1994, 60, 163-7.

[78] Li, TL; Lu, YB; Tian, ZK; Liu, LJ. Chang Bai Chai Hu zhong Chai Hu zaodai a dui xiaoshu shiyanxing gansunshang baohu zuoyong de shiyan yanjiu [Experimental study on protective effect on mouse hepatic injury caused by saikosaponin a from Bupleurum komarovianum Lincz.]. ACTA *Chinese Medicine and Pharmacology.*, 1988(1), 45.

[79] Chen, MF; Huang, CC; Liu, PS; Chen, CH; Shiu, LY. The proliferation and migration of hepatic stellate cells (HSCs) profoundly impact the pathogenesis of liver inflammation and fibrogenesi. *J Med Food.*, 2013, 16(9), 793-800. Epub, 2013/09/21.

[80] Chen, NL; Gu, F; Jia, KM; Peng, XJ; Deng, YL; Wang, GL. Xiao Chai Hu Tang dui 26 li yi xing, ding xing gan yan chong die gan ran zhi liao de tan tao [Study on treatment of 26 hepatitis B and D infections by minor bupleurum decoction]. *Zhonghua Nei Ke Za Zhi.*, 1990, 29(3), 144-6.

[81] Wu, YS. Chai Hu fang ji yao li xue yan jiu jin zhan [Study on pharmacology of Bupleurum-containing formulae]. *Suzhou Yi Xue.*, 1986, 9(1), 39-41.

[82] Sakae, A; Masakane, H; Yukio, O; Yasuhiko, O; Kenji, F; Hiroshi, O; et al. Treatment of chronic liver injury in mice by oral administration of xiao-chai-hu-tang. *J Ethnopharmacol.*, 1989, 25(2), 181-7.
[83] Chen, QL; Zheng, XY; Huang, XP. Chai Hu paozhipin dui xiaobaishu shiyanxing gansunshang de yingxiang [Influence on mouse hepatic injury by preparations of Radix Bupleuri]. *Zhong Cheng Yao.*, 1994, 16(3), 22-3.
[84] Wang, B-J; Liu, C-T; Tseng, C-Y; Wu, C-P; Yu, Z-R. Hepatoprotective and antioxidant effects of Bupleurum kaoi Liu (Chao et Chuang) extract and its fractions fractionated using supercritical CO2 on CCl4-induced liver damage. *Food Chem Toxicol.*, 2004, 42(4), 609-17.
[85] Zeng, XL; Xiao, JC; Hu, BR. Chai Hu dui xiangansuan huanhuamei de yingxiang [Influence on adenylate cyclase by Radix Bupleurum]. *Zhong Yao Yao Li Yu Lin Chuang.*, 1989, 5(1), 32-3.
[86] Lin, MD; Zeng, XL; Hu, BR. Chai Hu fenli zufen dui xiangansuan huanhuamei de yingxiang (2) [The effects of the isolated fractions from Bupleurum chinese DC on adenylate cyclase (2)]. *Zhong Yao Yao Li Yu Lin Chuang.*, 1991, 7(4), 17-20.
[87] Kok, LDS; Wong, CK; Leung, SF; Tsang, SF; Fung, KP; Choy, YM. Activation of the anti-tumor effector cells by Radix Bupleuri. *Immunopharmacology.*, 1995, 30(1995), 79-87.
[88] Cheng, Y-L; Chang, W-L; Lee, S-C; Liu, Y-G; Lin, H-C; Chen, C-J; et al. Acetone extract of Bupleurum scorzonerifolium inhibits proliferation of A549 human lung cancer cells via inducing apoptosis and suppressing telomerase activity. *Life Sci.*, 2003, 73(18), 2383-94.
[89] Xiao, Jian, ZF. Chai Hu zaodai d de kangzhongliu zuoyong yanjiu [Study on anti-tumour by saikosaponin d]. *Guo Wai Yi Xue - Zhong Yi Zhong Yao Fen Ce.*, 1988, 10(1), 45.
[90] Hsu, Y-L; Kuo, P-L; Weng, T-C; Yen, M-H; Chiang, L-C; Lin, C-C. The antiproliferative activity of saponin-enriched fraction from Bupleurum Kaoi is through Fas-dependent apoptotic pathway in human non-small cell lung cancer A549 cells. *Biol Pharm Bull.*, 2004, 27(7), 1112-5.
[91] Yao, M; Yang, J; Cao, L; Zhang, L; Qu, S; Gao, H. Saikosaponind inhibits proliferation of DU145 human prostate cancer cells by inducing apoptosis and arresting the cell cycle at G0/G1 phase. *Mol Med Rep.*, 2014, 10(1), 365-72. Epub, 2014/04/17.
[92] Tatsuta, M; Iishi, H; Baba, M; Nakaizumi, A; Uehara, H. Inhibition by xiao-chai-hu-tang (TJ-9) of development of hepatic foci induced by N-

nitrosomorpholine in Sprague-Dawley rats. *Jpn J Cancer Res.*, 1991, 82(9), 987-92.

[93] Kang, SJ; Lee, YJ; Kim, BM; Kim, YJ; Woo, HD; Jeon, HK; et al. Effect of Bupleuri Radix extracts on the toxicity of 5-fluorouracil in HepG2 hepatoma cells and normal human lymphocytes. *Basic Clin Pharmacol Toxicol.*, 2008, 103(4), 305-13.

[94] Li, JF. Gan Cao, Chai Hu, Ren Shen zhong de zaodai jiqi yanshengwu dui meihuoxing yingxiang de yanjiu [Study on activities of enzyme by saponins and its derivants from Radix Glycyrrhizae, Radix Bupleuri and Radix Ginseng]. *Zhong Cheng Xin Yao Yu Lin Chuang Yao Li.*, 1994, 5(4), 55-7.

[95] Sun, SX. Jizhong zhongyao jiere zuoyong zhi yaoli yanjiu [Parmacological study on antipyretic effects of several Chinese herbal medicine]. *Zhonghua Yi Xue Za Zhi.*, 1956(10), 964-8.

[96] Sun, H-X. Haemolytic activities and adjuvant effect of Bupleurum chinense saponins on the immune responses to ovalbumin in mice. *Vaccine.*, 2006, 24(9), 1324-31.

[97] Lu, BZ; Wu, ZC; Shan, JR; Xu, YJ. Chai Hu he Zhu Ling duotang de shenghua zuoyong ji kangfushe sunshang yuanli de yanjiu [Study on biochemical and antiradiation effects of bupleurum and polyporus polysaccharides]. *Jie Fang Jun Yi Xue Za Zhi.*, 1984, 9(1), 9-11.

[98] Dai, J; Ma, H; Fan, J; Li, Y; Wang, J; Ni, H; et al. Crude polysaccharide from an anti-UVB cell clone of Bupleurum scorzonerifolium protect HaCaT cells against UVB-induced oxidative stress. *Cytotechnology.*, 2011, 63(6), 599-607.

[99] Yang, XY; Ma, SP; Qu, R. Chai Hu tiquwu dui manxing yingji yiyu dashu zhizhi guoyanghua ji linba xibao zengzhi de yingxiang [Effects of Bupleurum chinense extracts on lipid peroxidation in chronic unpredictable mild stress model of depression in rats and lymphocyte proliferation in mice]. *J Chin Pharmaceut Univ.*, 2007, 38(5), 442-5.

[100] Gao, X; Zheng, X; Li, Z; Zhou, Y; Sun, H; Zhang, L; et al. Metabonomic study on chronic unpredictable mild stress and intervention effects of Xiaoyaosan in rats using gas chromatography coupled with mass spectrometry. *J Ethnopharmacol.*, 2011, 137(1), 690-9. Epub, 2011/07/02.

[101] Li, ZY; Guo, Z; Liu, YM; Liu, XM; Chang, Q; Liao, YH; et al. Neuroprotective effects of total saikosaponins of Bupleurum yinchowense on corticosterone-induced apoptosis in PC12 cells. *J Ethnopharmacol.*, 2013, 148(3), 794-803. Epub, 2013/05/23.

[102] Lee, B; Yun, HY; Shim, I; Lee, H; Hahm, DH. Bupleurum falcatum prevents depression and anxiety-like behaviors in rats exposed to repeated restraint stress. *J Microbiol Biotechnol.*, 2012, 22(3), 422-30. Epub, 2012/03/28.

[103] Yu, J-Q; Deng, A-J; Wu, L-Q; Zhang, Z-H; Liu, Y; Wang, W-J; et al. Osteoclast-inhibiting saikosaponin derivatives from Bupleurum chinense. *Fitoterapia.*, 2013, 85(0), 101-8.

[104] Chen, SM; Sato, N; Yoshida, M; Satoh, N; Ueda, S. Effects of Bupleurum scorzoneraefolium, Bupleurum falcatum, and saponins on nephrotoxic serum nephritis in mice. *J Ethnopharmacol.*, 2008, 116(3), 397-402.

[105] Lin, CC; Lin, LT; Yen, MH; Cheng, JT; Hsing, CH; Yeh, CH. Renal protective effect of xiao-chai-hu-tang on diabetic nephropathy of type 1-diabetic mice. *Evid Based Complement Alternat Med.*, 2012, 2012, 984024.

[106] Hao, Y; Piao, X; Piao, X. Saikosaponin-d inhibits beta-conglycinin induced activation of rat basophilic leukemia-2H3 cells. *Int Immunopharmacol.*, 2012, 13(3), 257-63. Epub, 2012/05/15.

[107] Chang, H-M; But, PP-H. Pharmacology and applications of Chinese materia medica. Singapore: World Scientific Publishing, 1986.

[108] Di, Yuan, XF. Chai Hu ji yizhi leiguchun jisu fuzuoyong de xiaoguo [Effects of Bupleurum-containing formula on side effects caused by steroid hormone]. *Guo Wai Yi Xue - Zhong Yi Zhong Yao Fen Ce.*, 1989, 11(1), 50.

[109] Lee, J-J; Kim, T; Cho, W-K; Ma, JY. Antithrombotic and antiplatelet activities of Soshiho-tang extract. *BMC Complement Altern Med.*, 2013, 13(1), 137.

[110] Testai, L; Silvio, C; Ammar, B; Luisa, P; Vincenzo, C; Martinotti, E. Vasorelaxant effects of the chloroformic crude extract of Bupleurum fruticosum L. (Umbelliferae) roots on rat thoracic aorta. *J Ethnopharmacol.*, 2005, 96(1-2), 93-7.

[111] Dong, L; Zhang, J. Chai Hu zhusheye zhi guominxing xiaochuan yili [A case of asthma caused by injection of Radix Bupleuri]. *Shanxi Zhong Yi.*, 1993, 14(2), 77.

[112] Tian, ZK; Ma, YL; Liu, LJ; An, FT; Wang, XK; Wang, L; et al. Chang Bai Chai Hu zaodai chengfen yanjiu [Study on saponins from Bupleurum komarovianum Lincz.]. *J Shenyang College Pharm.*, 1993, 10(2), 82-4, 93.

[113] Yang, Y. Chai Hu yinqi guomin fanying yili baogao [Report on a case of allergic reaction by Radix Bupleuri]. *Guizhou Yi Yao.*, 1991, 15(5), 306.
[114] Zhang, LY. Jizhu Chai Hu zhi guominxing xiuke yili [A case of allergic shock with intramuscular injection of Radix Bupleuri]. *Zhongguo Zhong Yao Za Zhi.*, 1993, 18(4), 246.
[115] Lu, ZH; Che, XK. Ji zhu Chai Hu zhi guo min xing xiu ke er li [Two cases of allergic shock with intramuscular injection of Radix Bupleuri]. *Zhongguo Zhong Yao Za Zhi.*, 1993, 18(4), 245.
[116] Chen, Y; Wang, J; Yuan, L; Zhou, L; Jia, X; Tan, X. Interaction of the main components from the traditional Chinese drug pair Chaihu-Shaoyao based on rat intestinal absorption. *Molecules.*, 2011, 16(11), 9600-10. Epub, 2011/11/19.
[117] Cheng, Y; Huang, Y; Tian, Y; Xu, L; Liu, GQ; Zahng, ZJ. Assessment of the effects of Radix bupleuri and vinegar-baked Radix bupleuri on cytochrome 450 activity by a six-drug cocktail approach. *Chin J Nat Med.*, 2013, 11(3), 302-8. Epub, 2013/06/04.
[118] Lee, C-H; Wang, J-D; Chen, P-C. Risk of liver injury associated with Chinese herbal products containing Radix Bupleuri in 639,779 patients with hepatitis B virus infection. *PLoS One.*, 2011, 6(1).
[119] Natural, Medicines, Comprehensive, Database. Bupleurum. [Internet]: Therapeutic Research Faculty, 2014 [updated Nov 1; cited, 2014 Nov 1]; Available from: http://naturaldatabase.therapeuticresearch.com/nd/Search.aspx?cs=&s=ND&pt=100&id=650&ds=&name=Chai+Hu+(BUPLEURUM)&searchid=49604084.
[120] Ikarashi, Y; Yuzurihara, M; Sakakibara, I; Takahashi, A; Ishimaru, H, Maruyama, Y. Effects of an oriental herbal medicine, "Saiboku-to", and its constituent herbs on Compound 48/80-induced histamine release from peritoneal mast cells in rats. *Phytomedicine.*, 2001, 8(1), 8-15.
[121] Huang, KC. The pharmacology of Chinese herbs. USA: CRC Press, 1999.
[122] Ishizaki, T; Sasaki, F; Ameshima, S; Shiozaki, K; Takahashi, H; Abe, Y; et al. Pneumonitis during interferon and/or herbal drug therapy in patients with chronic active hepatitis. *Eur Respir J.*, 1996, 9, 2691-6.
[123] Wu, J. Chai Hu, Ban Lan Gen zhusheye hunhe jizhu yinqi guominxing xiuke yili [A case of allergic shock with intramuscular administration of mixed injection of Radix Bupleuri and Radix Isatidis]. *Guangxi Zhong Yi Yao.*, 1993, 16(2), 28.

[124] Yue, FX. Chai Hu yu Qing Da Mei Su heyong zhi guominxing xiuke yili [A case of allergic shock with mixed injection of Radix Bupleuri and Gentamicin]. *Sichuan Yi Xue.*, 1991, 12(4), 247.
[125] Fugh, B-A. Herb-drug interactions. *Lancet.*, 2000, 9198(355).
[126] Therapeutic Goods Administration. Approved terminology for medicines. Woden, ACT: Commonwealth Department of Health and Aged Care, 1999.
[127] Medicines and Healthcare Products Regulatory Agency. Prohibited or restricted herbal ingredients. [Internet]: Medicines and Healthcare Products Regulatory Agency, 2011 [updated May 13; cited, 2014 Nov 1]; Available from: http://www.mhra.gov.uk/Howweregulate/Medicines/Herbalmedicinesregulation/Prohibitedorrestrictedherbalingredients/index.htm.
[128] The Pharmacopoeia Commission of People's Republic of China, editor. Zhonghua Ren Min Gong He Guo yao dian [Pharmacopoeia of the People's Republic of China]. Beijing: Chemical Industry Press, 2000.
[129] Government of Hong Kong. *Chinese Medicine* Ordinance Chapter 549. [Internet]: Bilingual Laws Information System, 1999 [updated June 8; cited, 2014 Nov 1]; Available from: http://www.legislation.gov.hk/blis_ind.nsf/e1bf50c09a33d3dc482564840019d2f4/75693bae1ea33cd3482567fa00292a6a?OpenDocument.

In: Chinese Herbs and Herbal Medicine
Editor: Brian L. Duke
ISBN: 978-1-63482-085-1
© 2015 Nova Science Publishers, Inc.

Chapter III

Chinese Herbal Medicines for Atopic Dermatitis: A Systematic Review

***Lu Li*[1,3], *Kam Lun Hon*[2], *Chi Chiu Wang*[3] and *Ping Chung Leung*[1,4]**

[1]Institute of Chinese Medicine, The Chinese University of Hong Kong, Shatin, New Territories, Hong Kong
[2]Departments of Paediatrics, The Chinese University of Hong Kong, Prince of Wales Hospital, Shatin, New Territories, Hong Kong
[3]Department of Obstetrics and Gynaecology, The Chinese University of Hong Kong, Shatin, New Territories, Hong Kong
[4]State Key Laboratory of Phytochemistry and Plant Resources in West China, The Chinese University of Hong Kong, Shatin, New Territories, Hong Kong

Abstract

Atopic dermatitis (AD) is a common chronic inflammatory skin disease in children that could adversely affect their quality of life, and its prevalence is increasing in the last few decades. As definitive cure is lacking, there has been a considerable interest on using traditional Chinese Herbal Medicines (CHM) as an alternative treatment for AD.

However, no data are available to provide an overview of the use of CHM for AD. In this chapter, we explored all the available relevant literatures on the clinical applications of CHM for AD, including its indications, contraindications, individual medicines, formulae, regimes, effectiveness, efficacy, safety, adverse effects and toxicity. The main objective is to review the available clinical studies on CHM for its therapeutic use in AD patients and the potential adverse outcomes. Over 140 literatures were identified, including the observational designed studies (exploratory studies, descriptive studies and analytical studies as case series, cohort studies, case-control studies, cross-sectional studies), the experimental studies (quasi- and randomized controlled trials) and the qualitative studies. Based on the principles and workflows from Centre for Evidence-Based Medicine of Oxford University and Cochrane Review, only few studies were selected for the systematic review and further meta-analysis. The result showed that compared with modern medicine groups, combined use of CHMs and modern medicines was significantly effective as a treatment option for atopic dermatitis. However there was insufficient proof on its safety although no specific safety problem was reported in the clinical trials. More scientific evidences through comprehensive studies on the efficacy and safety of CHM for AD are still necessary for its wider application.

Introduction

Atopic Dermatitis (AD)

Atopic dermatitis (AD), is a chronically relapsing inflammatory skin disease commonly associated with inhalant allergy [1]. The quality of life of patients could be adversely affected [2], as they are mostly suffering from dry and scaly skin with intensely itchy red, splotchy lesions in the bends of arms, legs, face, and neck [3]. Typical onsets of the disease occur in the children under five years of age in about 90% of patients. About 15% of schoolchildren aged 13 to 14 years have had a past history of AD [4].

The condition improves in most patients before adulthood, but it is also reported that 1–3% of adults in industrialized countries [5] suffer from AD. The incidence has increased two to three folds since the 1970s, with a slight female preponderance [6]. Based on a prediction made by a German research group in 2010, the probability of the incidence of AD among adults was 21.4% and for recurrence and persistence, up to 81.7% and 87.6% respectively [7].

AD, as a preexisting skin condition, may improve but usually worsen during pregnancy [8]. Some of the common modern therapies are advised to be avoided at any stage of pregnancy since they may have adverse effects on both the mothers and the fetuses. For example, systemic steroids can increase the risk of pregnancy-induced hypertension, pre-eclampsia, gestational diabetes, preterm labor, low birth weight and fetal malformations, such as cleft lip and palate [9].

Pathogenesis of AD

Pathogenesis of AD involves complex interactions between susceptible genes (filaggrin genes), immunological factors (immunoglobulin E, eosinophils, T helper cells, chemokines), skin barrier defects, infections, neuroendocrine factors (brain derived neurotrophic factor) and environmental factors (weather change, food and aeroallergens) [10, 11]. Major components in immune dysregulation include Langerhans' cells, inflammatory dendritic epidermal cells, monocytes, macrophages, lymphocytes, mast cells and keratinocytes. All of these components interact through an intricate cascade of cytokines leading to a predominance of Th2 cells [11] Th2 cytokines, interleukins IL-4, IL-5, IL-10 and IL-13, increase in the skin while there is a corresponding decrease in Th1 cytokines, mainly interferon-g and IL-2 Changes in the epidermis are attributed to the xerotic skin in the AD patient. Essential fatty acids (EFAs) are important components of the epidermis. Loss of EFAs results in increased transepidermal water loss and subsequent xerosis (dryness). Defects in the epidermal barrier also lead to increased susceptibility to allergens such as house dusts, mites, grass or pollen. When such allergens are in contact with susceptible skin, they stimulate Th2 lymphocytes to produce cytokines such as IL-4, IL-5 and IL-13 which in turn promote an increase in IgE synthesis [2, 12, 13]. AD patients often have high levels of IgE antibodies in response to house dusts mites and other allergens [14, 15].

AD patients also often have defective cell-mediated immunity, which is attributed to increased susceptibility to many bacterial, viral and fungal infections of the skin[2]. Certain factors, including Staphylococcus aureus colonization, stress, anxiety, systemic illness and xerosis, exacerbate or trigger AD[2].

Theory and Principle of CHM for AD

Modern drugs are developed to antagonize pathological targets or eliminate pathogenetic factors [16]. They may target on specific molecular changes in the body through specific molecular sites. Unlike this modern physiological model which is mainly concerned with different organs and tissues, the Chinese Medicine model is more concerned with bodily functions. Chinese Medicine focuses more on the body's response to pathogenetic factors and during the treatment processes using Chinese herbal medicines, the body's overall reactions rather than the isolated responses. The true value and strength of Chinese Medicine might occur in the strengthening of the recipients own vital energy so that his/her body may succeed in self-healing, through an enhanced defense and recovery ability [17].

According to the Chinese Medicine theory [18], Qi can be disrupted by "wind", "coldness", "summer-heat", "dampness", "dryness" or "fire evils". The main pathogenic factors of eczema are thought to be "wind", "dampness" and "heat". The mainly affected organs are "Spleen", "Kidney" and "Liver". The major causes of atopic dermatitis include "Spleen Deficiency", "Blood Heat and Dryness", "Dampness and Heat", "Kidney Deficiency" and "Liver Stasis". The diagnosis and treatment are based on the different causes and varied a lot among different patients. In Chinese Medicine, atopic dermatitis is considered not only a problem of the skin, but also reflects an imbalance of multi-systems in the body. So besides the medications to be applied to the skin with pathological changes, some other Chinese herbal medicines are required to improve the general health and physiological balance of the patients. For example, Radix Astragali (Huang Qi) is used to improve the immune system. Herbs such as Cortex Moutan Radix (Dan Pi), Radix Paeoniae Alba (Bai Shao), Potentilla Chinensis Ser (Wei Ling Cai) and Radix Glycyrrhizae (Gan Cao) are common choices for the treatment of allergy [19].

Chinese herbal medicines are combined as formulae to enhance the therapeutic functions of individual herbs which as a result, work together to create a more harmonious effect on the body as a systemic treatment for disorders [20]. Modern therapeutics, containing pure chemicals only, are usually administered singly although combined therapeutic cocktails are recommended from time to time. Presumably each individual Chinese herbs either singly or combined, and containing numerous chemicals, may achieve synergistic effects inside the body, thus delivering unique therapeutic functions. The pharmacological effects of each individual Chinese herb may not be representative of the final therapeutic function of the formula.

Interactions exist amongst active components within an individual Chinese herb as well as between the components of a formula [21]. Chinese herbal medicine therefore archives its therapeutic effects in a unique way different from Modern medicine.

Current Treatments for AD

There is no guaranteed cure for AD so far. Management of this condition includes use of emollient, topical and systemic antimicrobial agents, corticosteroid or immunomodulating agents [2]. Corticosteroids (CS), either in the topical or systemic form, remain the gold standard of treatment for AD [23]. However, CS has a wide range of immunomodulatory effects, such as the suppression of cytokine production, adhesion molecule expression and leukocyte chemotaxis [24]. CS is also associated with deranged metabolism, growth suppression and increased susceptibility to infections. In particular, the use of potent topical CS in AD may cause significant suppression of the hypothalamicpituitary - adrenal axis [25]. The alternative treatment by tacrolimus or pimecrolimus has a potentially elevated risk in cancer [26], whereas skin atrophy is the mostly seen adverse reaction with CS [27]. More specific immunomodulatory agents (e.g. topical tacrolimus) are available [28]. However, some patients remain symptomatic and may seek other complementary treatment.

Various dietary therapies including the use of Chinese herbs are popular among the patients in Asia [29]. In the early 1990s, a Chinese medicine decoction (Zemaphyte) was found to be efficacious for the treatment of AD in both children [30, 31] and adults [32] in the U.K. Traditional Chinese herbal medicine (CHM) since then has been considered an alternative and possibly promising therapy in the treatment of AD.

Objectives

Although Chinese herbal medicine has been widely used in many Asian countries for centuries and has enjoyed early studied as an alternative and complement therapy for atopic dermatitis in Europe, its beneficial effects on children with AD have not been consistently demonstrated while undesirable side effects have been noted. A limited number of clinical trials using Chinese

Medicine in children and adults with AD did not show convincing results [33, 34, 35, 36], and the latest systematic reviews by Cochrane group reported that no conclusive evidence could support that Chinese herbal medicines taken by mouth or applied topically to the skin could reduce the severity of eczema in children or adults.

In this chapter, we will give an overview of Chinese herbal medicine as a treatment for atopic dermatitis, emphasising its efficacy and safety.

Clinical Applications

We carried out a literature survey on the use of Chinese herbal medicines for the treatments of atopic dermatitis in the recent ten years (2005-2014) in the following databases: Cochrane Central Register of Controlled Trials, mainly Cochrane Database of Systematic Reviews and Cochrane Database of Abstracts of Reviews of Effects; EMBASE; Cumulative Index to Nursing and Allied Health Literature (CINAHL); Chinese Biomedical Database (CBM); Medline (and PreMedline); PubMed; China Journal Net (CJN); China National Knowledge Infrastructure (CNKI); Wiley Inter Science and Wan Fang Database (Chinese Ministry of Science & Technology), with the key words "atopic dermatitis" and/or "eczema" and "Chinese medicine" and/or "Chinese therapy". Up to 20 Nov, 2014, 315 related studies were identified (Figure 1). Most of the literatures were obtained from CNKI, CJN and WanFang databases. And most of the literatures (74.5%) were published in only Chinese whilst some of the Chinese literatures (25.5%) provided English abstracts. After further exclusion of animal studies (23.5%), genetic studies (20.6%), chemical studies (7.3%) and microbiology studies (4.1%), in total 141 (44.8%) clinical studies of Chinese medicines for recurrent miscarriage were included for further selection (Figure 1).

Based on the principles and workflows provided by the Centre for Evidence-Based Medicine of Oxford University and Cochrane Review, we further excluded the commentary articles (19.9%), case reports (11.3%) and other review articles (7.8%). The sample size was usually very small in case reports, mostly 2-6 participants, and the details of Chinese herbal medicine intervention varied a lot, so the case reports can hardly represent the general application of Chinese herbal medicines. The commentary articles only focused on the theory and principles of Chinese herbal medicines for atopic dermatitis. Other review articles only gave summaries and conclusions on the clinical topics, without systematically reviewing the clinical trials. The remaining 86 clinical trials were selected for this systematic review (Figure 1).

After further excluding the 48 case series and the 28 and 4 studies reported in two Cochrane reviews [37, 38], 6 randomized controlled trials [39, 40, 41, 42, 43, 44] were included for further meta-analysis in the present study(Figure 1). Other studies, like cohort studies, case-control studies, cross-sectional studies, quasi-randomized controlled trials and qualitative studies were not identified.

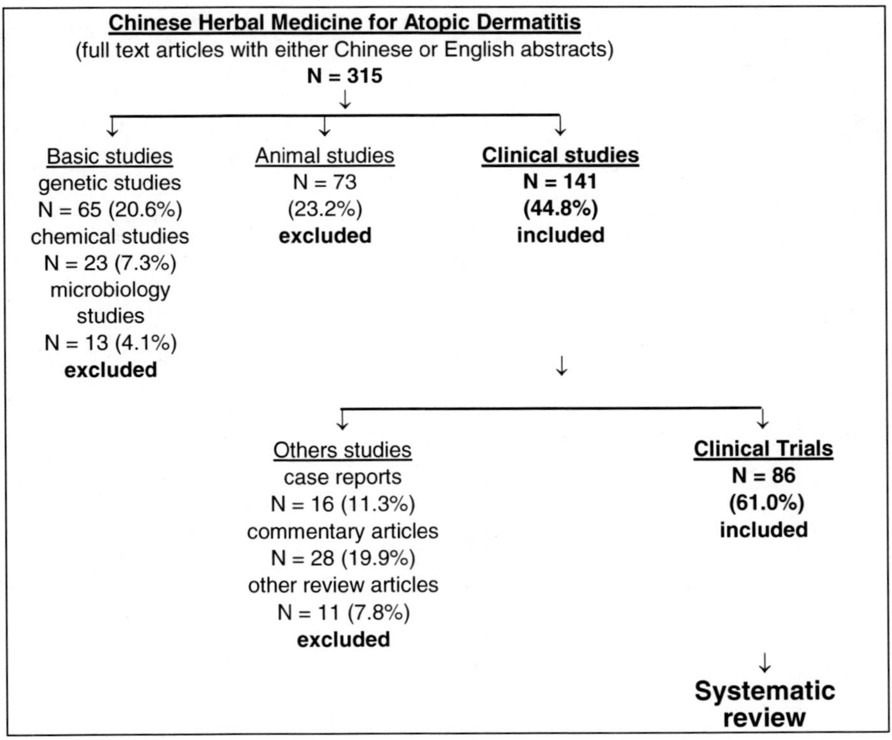

Figure 1. Study inclusions and exclusions for systematic review.

Common CHM for AD

Amongst all the formulae applied as treatments for atopic dermatitis in these 86 clinical trials, over 30 formulae were reported.

Table 1. Top 5 most common individual CHMs for AD from literatures

Order	English Name	Biological Name	Chinese Name	Frequency*	Daily mean dose± SEM[a] (g)	Recommended dose[b] (g)	Therapeutic actions[c]
1	Milkvetch Root	*Radix Astragali*	Huang Qi	59.3%	19.6±1.01	9-30	Regulate "Qi" & "Blood", Remove "Damp"
2	Largehead Atractylodes Rhizome	*Rhizoma Atractylodis Macrocephalae*	Bai Zhu	54.7%	16.7±1.13	6-12	Regulate "Qi" & "Blood"
3	Liquorice Root Radix Et Rhizoma	Liquorice Root *Radix Et Rhizoma*	Gan Cao	40.7%	7.4±0.77	2-10	Remove "Heat"
4	Chinese Angelica Radix Angelicae	Chinese Angelica *Radix Angelicae*	Dang Gui	34.9%	15.1±1.21	6-12	Supplement and regulate "Blood"
5	Swordlike Atractylodes Rhizome	*Atractlodis Rhizoma*	Cang Zhu	29.1%	10.2±0.80	3-9	Remove "Heat" & "Damp"

* Frequency = number of literature of each CHM/total amount of literatures * 100

a Daily mean dose is referred to the mean of the reported daily dose in all included clinical trials.

b Recommended dose is referred to the dose range of each CHM in "Chinese Pharmacopeia"

c Functions of the individual CHM as treatment for AD.

Some formulae were prescribed and modified basing on the principle of some well-known classical formulae, the experience of Chinese medicine practitioners as well as the clinical presentations of the individual patients. It is not possible to define the most commonly used formulae, and even the more popular formulae were modified freely by the clinicians involved who mainly worked on the basic principles of: 1) improving the function of "Spleen", like "Jianpi Decoction" [45]; 2) stabilising and regulating the circulation, like "Liangxue Fangfeng Decoction" [44] and "Danggui Decoction" [41]; 3) removing the "Dampness" of the body, like "Lishi Decoction" [42]; 4) relieving the "Heat", like "Huanglian Decoction" [46], etc.

The top five most commonly used individual Chinese herbal medicines (Table 1) included Radix Astragali (Huang Qi) and Rhizoma atractylodis macrocephalae (Bai Zhu), (for the balance of the immune system); Radix glycyrrhizae (Gan Cao) (for the removal of "heat" and maintenance of internal harmony); Radix angelicae sinensis (Dang Gui) (for the regulation of blood circulation); Rhizoma atractylodis (Cang Zhu) (for the clearance of "damp-heat"). Many pharmacological studies have reported anti-allergic, anti-inflammatory, anti-itching and sedative effects of these herbs [47].

Efficacy and Effectiveness

Summary of Previous Studies

In the early 1990s, Sheehan's team carried out a randomized placebo-controlled double-blind trial of a specific prescription (Zemaphyte) for widespread non-exudative atopic eczema [30] and reported that it was efficacious for the treatment of AD in both children [31] and adults [32] in the UK. The conclusion was that Chinese medicinal medicines have a therapeutic potential in treating eczema and other skin diseases. However, Zemaphyte has been withdrawn from the market since 2004 and a subsequent randomized placebo-controlled, cross-over trial of the same decoction by a group of dermatologists failed to demonstrate the beneficial effects on Chinese patients with recalcitrant AD in Hong Kong [48].

A five herb formula (PHF) decoction, developed by our team in Hong Kong, has been proved well-tolerated, gave only minor side effects and was effective on improving the quality of life and reducing the need for topical GC in children and adolescents. Bench studies also demonstrated that there are favorable immunomodulatory effects [49, 50]. There are many different Chinese herbal medicine formulae that have been studied as AD treatments in recent years, such as Shuangfujin formula for acute eczema [51] and a Kampo formula for Kikyo patients with AD [52]. In our previous review in 2011 [53], we have summarised the relevant clinical studies by different study types, including randomised controlled trials, case reports and series and laboratory studies, on both effectiveness and safety of the Chinese medicine formulae.

Another systematic review on the topic of Chinese herbal medicine for AD was by Zhang's team in Cochrane Review Group [35], which located the relevant clinical trials from 1980 to 2004, but only four small poorly reported RCTs of the same product, Zemaphyte, were found and the results were heterogeneous. In their updated study in 2013 [37], the literature search year has been extended from 1946 to 2012, and 28 clinical trials were included for the review.

However, the conclusion was that no reliable evidence could be provided for the therapeutic efficacy of CHM for the treatment of AD.

Updates on Efficacy and Effectiveness

In our study, the general effective rate of Chinese herbal medicines for atopic dermatitis in all 86 clinical trials was noted. The efficacy ranged from 56.7% to 96.7%. Over 75.9% of the studies exceeded 70% effective rate, 62.1% exceeded 80% and 20.7% exceeded 90%. The daily doses of individual Chinese herbal medicines ranged from 5g to 30g.

To assess the effectiveness of Chinese herbal medicines for atopic dermatitis, after further selections (Figure 1) by excluding the 48 case series and the 28 and 4 studies reported in two Cochrane review [35, 37], 6 randomized controlled trials were included for a further analysis in comparing the effectiveness between Chinese herbal medicines and other approaches for atopic dermatitis. Other approaches included modern medicines alone and combined Chinese herbal medicines and modern medicines.

Amongst these clinical trials, no placebo controlled trial was found. The comparisons on the effectiveness were all between combined Chinese herbal medicine and modern medicine group and western medicine alone group.

The recorded modern medicines included Cetirizine Dihydrochloride, Loratadine Tablet, Mepivacaine Hydrochloride and Adrenaline Injection, Ethacridine Lactate, Acrivastine Capsules, Mometasone Furoate cream and Hydrocortisone Butyrate Cream.

	Combined Medicines		Western Medicines			Risk Ratio	
Study or Subgroup	Events	Total	Events	Total	Weight	M-H, Random, 95% CI	Year
Zhang 2005	29	31	21	30	19.6%	1.34 [1.04, 1.72]	2005
Li 2006	42	44	30	37	34.0%	1.18 [0.99, 1.39]	2006
Shi 2008	23	25	12	22	9.1%	1.69 [1.13, 2.51]	2008
Chen 2011	29	31	21	30	19.6%	1.34 [1.04, 1.72]	2011
Hu 2013	14	23	2	11	1.0%	3.35 [0.92, 12.23]	2013
Li 2014	27	31	21	31	16.8%	1.29 [0.97, 1.70]	2014
Total (95% CI)		185		161	100.0%	1.31 [1.15, 1.49]	
Total events	164		107				

Heterogeneity: $Tau^2 = 0.01$; $Chi^2 = 6.23$, df = 5 (P = 0.28); $I^2 = 20\%$
Test for overall effect: Z = 4.16 (P < 0.0001)

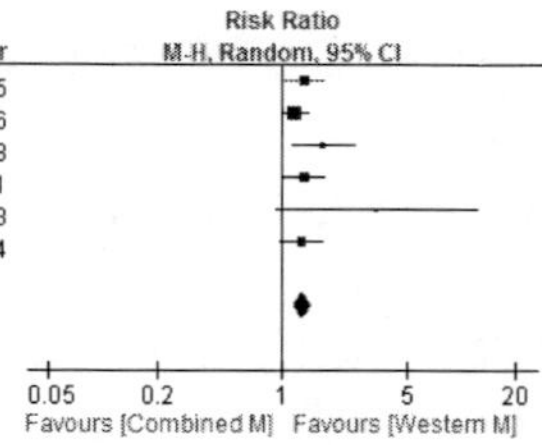

Figure 2. Comparison on effectiveness between combined medicines and modern medicines.

The meta-analysis of limited randomized controlled trials showed that the combined Chinese herbal medicines and modern medicines group enjoyed a significantly higher effectiveness rate than modern medicine alone group (relative risk=1.31; 95% confidence interval: 1.15–1.49; I2 = 20%; P<0.0001) (Figure 2), so it did support the assumption that combined medicines group were more effective than modern medicines alone.

Limitations and Difficulties

Most of the included clinical trials were written in Chinese. Although some of the publications provided English abstracts but in most cases English full texts are not available. This largely limited the supply of useful the information.

The Chinese reports are also of poor quality. Firstly, no placebo control studies were identified in our review. Secondly, information on the methodology was insufficient in many randomised controlled trials. For example, many trials only stated "randomization was applied", but no details of the randomization, allocation and concealment methods were provided. Thirdly, due to the insufficiency of data, further analysis for subgroups was not possible. For example, different Chinese herbal formulae were applied in many clinical trials, hence a further subgroup analysis basing on the Chinese Medicine theory of AD impossible. Therefore, any conclusion made on the effectiveness could only reflect the effects of Chinese herbal medicines used against a general understanding of atopic dermatitis, not specific to any traditional syndrome commonly referred to in Chinese Medicine.

Safety and Adverse Events

Current Knowledge on Safety

During the historical application and practice of Chinese herbal medicines, safety has been taken for granted if applied properly. Many Chinese Medicine practioners or herbal medicine experts strongly believe that the different formulae used for AD, were safe [53].

In Sheehan's clinical trial of Zemaphyte [30], there was no evidence of hematological, renal or hepatic toxicity. In Hon's placebo-controlled study [23], no clinical or biochemical evidence of any adverse drug reaction by PHF was found during the study period, and the capsules were well tolerated by the children. In Zhang's systematic review [37], some mild adverse effects were reported, like mild gastrointestinal symptoms, but none were regarded as serious.

As a matter of fact, Chinese herbal medicines are not totally free of risk. Some individual Chinese herbs have been reported to be potentially toxic. At least 31 Chinese herbs have been classified as toxic and contraindicated during pregnancy, which have been listed in the Chinese Pharmacopeia. Sometimes, the potential toxicity could be modified or eliminated with special means like modifications dosage adjustment and the change on the duration of treatment. However, scientific and systematic evidence that could confirm the safety of the Chinese herbs would need to be worked out [54, 55].

Adverse Outcomes

In this study, the occurrence of failure of treatment and adverse effects or toxicity of Chinese medicines during and after treatment were further reviewed and analysed. The 6 randomised clinical trials compared combined Chinese herbal medicine and modern medicine treatment with modern medicines treatment alone, and the results indicated that the intervention failure was significantly lower in the combined medicines group than in modern medicines group (relative risk=0.35; 95% confidence interval: 0.23-0.54; $I2 = 0\%$; $P<0.00001$) (Figure 3).

As to the adverse effects, Li's study (ref) reported that no side effects were observed during treatments, Shi's study (ref) reported that the laboratory examinations on blood, urine and stool tests and liver and kidney functions were all normal, and no adverse effects were observed after treatments. Others reports did not study the safety issue at all.

	Combined Medicines		Western Medicines			Risk Ratio	
Study or Subgroup	Events	Total	Events	Total	Weight	M-H, Random, 95% CI	Year
Zhang 2005	2	31	9	30	8.3%	0.22 [0.05, 0.91]	2005
Li 2006	2	44	7	37	7.6%	0.24 [0.05, 1.09]	2006
Shi 2008	2	25	10	22	8.8%	0.18 [0.04, 0.72]	2008
Chen 2011	2	31	9	30	8.3%	0.22 [0.05, 0.91]	2011
Hu 2013	9	23	9	11	51.3%	0.48 [0.27, 0.85]	2013
Li 2014	4	31	10	31	15.8%	0.40 [0.14, 1.14]	2014
Total (95% CI)		**185**		**161**	**100.0%**	**0.35 [0.23, 0.54]**	
Total events	21		54				

Heterogeneity: $Tau^2 = 0.00$; $Chi^2 = 3.88$, df = 5 (P = 0.57); $I^2 = 0\%$
Test for overall effect: Z = 4.89 (P < 0.00001)

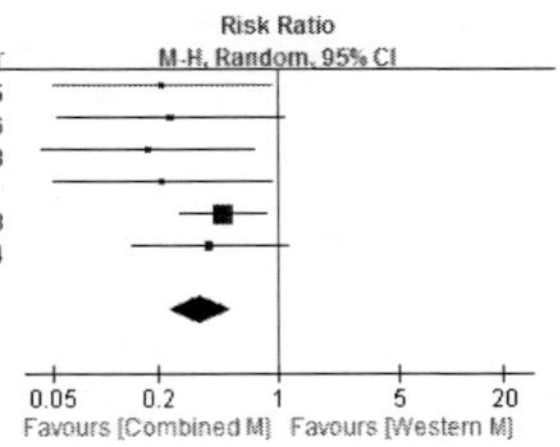

Figure 3 Comparison of failure of treatments between combined medicines and modern medicines.

Limitations and Difficulties

Study designs and clinical trial qualities again produced limitations and difficulties. Around 1/3 of the studies neither included nor monitored the adverse effects as outcome measures. It may be due to the lack of awareness on the safety issue of Chinese herbal medicines in general. In the Cochrane review [37], 24 in 28 studies did report the adverse outcomes, but only brief and descriptive information was provided. Further subgroup analysis to evaluate the different types of adverse outcomes became impossible. This limited us to draw an appropriate conclusion. We could only support that probably using Chinese herbal medicines for the treatment of atopic dermatitis is safe. Further studies and larger randomized placebo-controlled trials are needed to confirm the safety issue.

Conclusion and Recommendations

Chinese herbal medicines, as a promising alternative therapy for many disorders that could not be completely cured by modern medicines, have remained popular in many Asian countries and are apparently increasingly accepted worldwide today. In this chapter, we focused on one of its clinical application, atopic dermatitis, aiming to obtain and provide more evidences on the efficacy and safety of Chinese herbal treatment.

However, sufficient evidence to support the application of Chinese herbal medicines alone as a treatment for atopic dermatitis is not available, although meta-analysis showed that combined Chinese herbal medicines and modern medicines together has superior therapeutic and safety effects compared with modern medicines alone. Clinical studies on Chinese herbal medicines with higher quality in methodology and more large scales of randomized placebo-controlled trials are still needed.

Acknowledgments

L.L received the Hop Wai Scholarship and Zi Ying Scholarship from the Institute of Chinese Culture and Postgraduate Student Grants for Overseas Academic Activities from the Graduate School, The Chinese University of Hong Kong during herb PhD study, to receive the Cochrane Review training in Oxford University and Freiburg Conference; and in Liverpool Women's Hospital with the Cochrane Pregnancy and Childbirth Group. In 2013 and 2014, L.L. has received fellowships from Deutscher Akademischer AustauschDienst (DAAD), Research Fellowship Scheme (RFS) and National Natural Science Foundation of China (NSFC) Young Scientist Fund project for her research projects on Chinese herbal medicines in Germany, Hong Kong SAR China and Mainland China, respectively.

(Publications in our team are underlined)

References

[1] Leung DY. Atopic dermatitis: the skin as a window into the pathogenesis of chronic allergic diseases. *J. Allergy Clin. Immunol.,* 1995; 96:302-318.
[2] Leung AK, Hon KL, Robson WL. Atopic dermatitis. Adv Pediatr. 2007;54:241-73.
[3] Berke, R; Singh, A; Guralnick, M. "Atopic dermatitis: an overview". *American Family Physician,* 2012;86(1): 35–42.
[4] Leung R, Wong G, Lau J, Ho A, Chan JK, Choy D, Douglass C, Lai CK: Prevalence of asthma and allergy in Hong Kong schoolchildren: an ISAAC study. *Eur. Respir. J.,* 1997;10:354-360.
[5] Saito, Hirohisa. "Much Atopy about the Skin: Genome-Wide Molecular Analysis of Atopic Eczema". *Inte. Arch. Allergy Immunol.,* 2005;137 (4):319–325.

[6] The prevalence of atopic dermatitis in Oregon school children. *J. Am. Acad. Dermatol.,* 2000;43:649-655.

[7] Peters AS, Kellberger J, Vogelberg C, Dressel H, Windstetter D, Weinmayr G, Genuneit J, Nowak D, Mutius E, Radon K. Prediction of the incidence, recurrence, and persistence of atopic dermatitis in adolescence: a prospective cohort study. *J. Allergy Clin. Immunol.,* 2010;126(3):590-5.e1-3.

[8] Renner R, Sticherling M. Chronic inflammatory and autoimmune mediated dermatoses during pregnancy. Course and prognosis for mother and child. *Hautarzt,* 2010;61(12):1021-6.

[9] MA Belfort, GR Saade, MR, JP Phelan, GA Dildy. In: Critical Care Obstetrics. 5th ed. Hoboken, New Jersey, United States. Wiley-Blackwell. 2010:332.

[10] Leung AK, Barber KA: Managing childhood atopic dermatitis. *Adv. Ther.,* 2003;20:129-137.

[11] Leung DY, Bieber T: Atopic dermatitis. *Lancet,* 2003;361:151-160.

[12] Kondo H, Ichikawa Y, Imokawa G: Percutaneous sensitization with allergens through barrier-disrupted skin elicits a Th2-dominant cytokine response. *Eur. J. Immunol.,* 1998;28:769-779.

[13] Hon KL, Leung TF. Seromarkers in childhood atopic dermatitis. *Expert Rev. Dermatol.,* 2010;5:299-314.

[14] Hon KL, Leung TF, Ching G, Chow CM, Luk V, Ng PC. Patterns of food and aeroallergen sensitization in childhood eczema. *Acta Paediatr.,* 2008;97:1734-1737.

[15] Hon KL, Chan IH, Chow CM, Wang SS, Lam CW, Ng PC, Leung TF: Specific IgE of common foods in Chinese children with eczema. Pediatr Allergy Immunol 2011;22:50-53.

[16] Jiang WY. Therapeutic wisdom in traditional Chinese medicine: a perspective from modern science. *Trends in Pharmacological Sciences,* 2005;26(11): p. 558-563.

[17] Wang BC, Zhu LC, Chen Q. Primary study on the application of Serum Pharmacology in Chinese traditional medicine. *Colloids and Surfaces B-Biointerfaces,* 2005; 43(3-4): p. 194-197.

[18] Lin X, Tu C, Yang C. Study on treatment of eczema by Chinese herbal medicine with anti-type IV allergic activity. *Zhongguo Zhong Xi Yi Jie He Za Zhi,* 2000;20:258-260.

[19] Zhang EQ. In: Clinical of Traditional Chinese Medicine [II] Shanghai: Publishing House of Shanghai College of Traditional Chinese Medicine, 1990.

[20] Zhang JB. Jing Yue Quan Shu. Shanghai: Shanghai Science and Technology Press 1959.

[21] Judith X. Becerra, D.L.V., P. H. Evans, and W. S. Bowers Interactions Between Chemical and Mechanical Defenses in the Plant Genus Bursera and Their Implications for Herbivores Amer. Zool., 2001;41(4): p. 865-876.

[22] Hon KL, Chan CL, Leung PC. Chinese herbal medicine research in eczema treatment. *Chin. Med.,* 2011; 6:17.

[23] Hon KL, Leung TF, Wong Y, Lam WK, Guan DQ, Ma KC, Sung YT, Fok TF, Leung PC. A Pentaherbs Capsule as a Treatment Option for Atopic Dermatitis in Children: An Open-Labeled Case Series. *Am. J. Chin. Med.,* 2004;32:941–950.

[24] Pucci N, Lombardi E, Novembre E, Farina S, Bernardini R, Rossi E, Favilli T, Vierucci A: Urinary eosinophil protein ¡Ñ and serum eosinophil cationic protein in infants and young children with atopic dermatitis: correlation with disease activity. *J. Allergy Clin. Immunol.,* 2000;105:353-357.

[25] Ellison JA, Patel LM, Ray DW, David TJ, Clayton PE: Hypothalamic-pituitaryadrenal function and glucocorticoid sensitivity in atopic dermatitis. *Pediatrics,* 2000;105:794-799.

[26] Tennis P, Gelfand JM, Rothman KJ. Evaluation of cancer risk related to atopic dermatitis and use of topical calcineurin inhibitors. *Br. J. Dermatol.,* 2011;165:465-473.

[27] Korting HC, Unholzer A, Schäfer-Korting M, Tausch I, Gassmueller J, Nietsch KH. Different skin thinning potential of equipotent medium-strength glucocorticoids. *Skin Pharmacol. Appl. Skin Physiol.,* 2002;15: 85-91.

[28] Hon KL, Lam MC, Leung TF, Chow CM, Wong E, Leung AK: Assessing itch in children with atopic dermatitis treated with tacrolimus: objective versus subjective assessment. *Adv. Ther.,* 2007;24:23-28.

[29] Hon KL, Ma KC, Wong Y, Leung TF, Fok TF: A survey of traditional Chinese medicine use in children with atopic dermatitis attending a paediatric dermatology clinic. *J. Dermatolog. Treat.,* 2005;16:154-157.

[30] Sheehan MP, Atherton DJ. A controlled trial of traditional Chinese medicinal plants in widespread non-exudative atopic eczema. *Br. J. Dermatol.,* 1992;126:179–184.

[31] Sheehan MP, Atherton DJ. One-year follow up of children treated with Chinese medicinal herbs for atopic eczema. *Br. J. Dermatol.,* 1994; 130:488–493.

[32] Sheehan MP, Stevens H, Ostlere LS, Atherton DJ, Brostoff J, Rustin MH. Follow-up of adult patients with atopic eczema treated with Chinese herbal therapy for 1 year. *Clin. Exp. Dermatol.,* 1995;20:136–140.

[33] Fung AY, Look PC, Chong LY, But PP, Wong E: A controlled trial of traditional Chinese herbal medicine in Chinese patients with recalcitrant atopic dermatitis. *Int. J. Dermatol.,* 1999;38:387-392.

[34] Johnston G, Bilbao R, Graham-Brown RA: The use of complementary medicine in children with atopic dermatitis in secondary care in Leicester. *Br. J. Dermatol.,* 2003;149:566-571.

[35] Zhang W, Leonard T, Bath-Hextall F, Chambers CA, Lee C, Humphreys R, Williams HC: Chinese herbal medicine for atopic eczema. *Cochrane Database Syst. Rev.,* 2005, 2:CD002291.

[36] Hon KL, Leung AK: Powerful proprietary Chinese medicine for eczema? *Clin. Exp. Dermatol.,* 2010;35:e14-e15.

[37] Gu S, Yang AWH, Xue CCL, Li CG, Pang C, Zhang W, Williams HC. Chinese herbal medicine for atopic eczema. *Cochrane Database Syst. Rev.,* 2013;9:CD002291.

[38] Zhang W, Leonard T, Bath-Hextall F, Chambers CA, Lee C, Humphreys R, Williams HC: Chinese herbal medicine for atopic eczema. *Cochrane Database Syst. Rev.,* 2004;2:CD002291.

[39] Zhang YH, Chen BJ. Clinical observation on integrated medicines for AD. *Chinese Journal of Dermatovenereology of Integrate,* 2005;4(4): 207-210. [Chinese]

[40] Li F, Luo WH. Integrated medicines for 44 AD patients. *Hunan Journal of Traditional Chinese Medicine,* 2006;22(4):20-21. [Chinese]

[41] Shi YJ, Zhang CM, Ma DM, Liu Y, Zhang DM, Zhang CH, Wei G, Dong LY. Clinical Study on Treatment of Atopic Dermatitis by Integrated Traditional Chinese and Western Medicine. *Chinese Journal of Integrated Traditional and Western Medicine,* 2008;28(8):686-688. [Chinese]

[42] Chen BJ, Zhang YH. Study of Jianpi Lishi decoction as treatments for AD. *Jilin Journal of Traditional Chinese Medicine,* 2011;31(4):335-336. [Chinese]

[43] Luo YS, Zhang BX, Guo YP. Random control study on treating AD in the integrative medicine. *Clinical Journal of Chinese Medicine,* 2013;5 (3):10-12. [Chinese]

[44] Li L. Integrated medicines for AD treatments. *Neimenggu Chinese Medicine,* 2014;27:56-57. [Chinese]

[45] Jin PZ, Ye QH, Shen M. Observation of efficacy of Jianpi Zhiyang granules for 32 cases with atopic dermatitis. *Henan Traditional Chinese Medicine,* 2007;27(12):61-2.

[46] Xiao WM, Li G, Luo B, Zhu QJ. Observation of efficacy of Huailian decoction for atopic dermatitis. *Journal of China Traditional Chinese Medicine Information,* 2011;3(3):37–9.

[47] Huang TK: A Handbook of the Composition and Pharmacology of Common Chinese Drugs Beijing: Chinese Medicine and Technology Press. 1998.

[48] Fung AY, Look PC, Chong LY, But PP, Wong E: A controlled trial of traditional Chinese herbal medicine in Chinese patients with recalcitrant atopic dermatitis. *Int. J. Dermatol.,* 1999;38:387-392.

[49] Leung TF, Wong KY, Wong CK, Fung KP, Lam CW, Fok TF, et al. In vitro and clinical immunomodulatory effects of a novel Pentaherbs concoction for atopic dermatitis. *Br. J. Dermatol.,* 2008;158:1216–1223.

[50] Chan BC, Hon KL, Leung PC, Sam SW, Fung KP, LeeMY, et al. Traditional Chinesemedicine for atopic eczema: PentaHerbs formula suppresses inflammatory mediators release from mast cells. *J. Ethnopharmacol.,* 2008;120: 85-91.

[51] Bai YP, Yang DQ, Wang YM: Clinical study on treatment of acute eczema by Shuangfujin. *Zhongguo Zhong Xi Yi Jie He Za Zhi,* 2007;27: 72-75.

[52] Kobayashi H: Clinical evaluation of Hochuekkito in the treatment of atopic dermatitis: a multicenter, double-blind, randomized, placebocontrolled study. Nippon Yakurigaku Zasshi 2008;132:285-287.

[53] Hon KL, Chan BCL, Leung PC. Chinese herbal medicine research in eczema treatment. *Chinese Medicine,* 2011;6:17.

[54] Li L, Dou LX, Leung PC, Wang CC. Chinese herbal medicines for threatened miscarriage (Review). Cochrane Database of Systematic Reviews 2012, Issue 5. Art. No.: CD008510. DOI: 10.1002/14651858. CD008510.pub2.

[55] Li L, Dou LX, James P Neilson, Leung PC, Wang CC. Adverse outcomes of Chinese medicines used for threatened miscarriage: a systematic review and meta-analysis. *Human Reproduction Update,* 2012;18(5):504–524.

Index

A

B

D

E

H

I

J

K

L

M

N

O

P

T

U

V

W

Z